THAT'S A BUNCH OF QUACKERY!

How to Avoid Being Pick-Pocketed by Misleading Claims in the Fitness Industry

By

Jeanne "Bean" Murdock

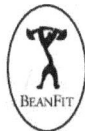

Copyright © Jeanne "Bean" Murdock 2016
BEANFIT Publishing
Paso Robles, CA
USA

Copyright © 2016 Jeanne "Bean" Murdock
Originally written and copyrighted in 1997.
All rights reserved.
This book may not be reproduced, in whole or in part,
including illustrations, in any form (beyond that copying
permitted by Sections 107 and 108 of the U.S. Copyright
Law and except by reviewers for the public press), without
written permission from the author.

Library of Congress Control Number: 2015920716
ISBN: 09770678-4-x
EAN: 978-09770678-4-8
The information, recommendations, instructions, and
advice contained in this book are intended for general
reference purposes only and are not intended to address
specific medical or dietary conditions or needs. This
information is not a substitute for professional medical or
nutritional advice or a medical exam. Prior to following any
advice, instructions, or recommendations in this book, and
prior to participating in any exercise or dietary program or
activity, you should seek the advice of your physician or
other qualified health professional. No information in this
book should be used to diagnose, treat, cure, or prevent any
medical or health condition.

All chapter photos were taken by Jeanne "Bean" Murdock

Cover image by Jim Tyler and edited by the author

I dedicate this book to everyone who cares enough about themselves to learn how to lead a healthy lifestyle *and* to practice it.

ACKNOWLEDGMENTS

Most of my thanks go to Joe who always reminded me to be patient and believe in my work.

Thanks to my friends and family, too, for not revealing my undercover alias.

Thanks to Dr. Griffin for reviewing the chiropractor section.

Thanks to Ralph La Forge who has been my health and fitness mentor my whole career, always available at a moment's notice, never asking for anything in return.

TABLE OF CONTENTS

FOREWORD

I have known Jeanne "Bean" Murdock for 20 give or take years. In no small way she practices what she teaches—and has dedicated herself to improving physical activity and fitness habits in individuals as well as large groups. Jeanne has written the Divine Comedy of dealing with anything beyond the sphere of no-nonsense exercise and fitness. I fully concur with her thesis. I think her ultimate message, which is also one that I am endeared to myself, is "Just move, and move often." As trite as it may sound, regular daily physical activity (of nearly any kind at even low-moderate intensity levels) reduces the unnecessary burden of chronic disease, especially diabetes and cardiovascular disease. Yes, there is abundant mythology and quackery throughout the fitness (and health care) industry; quick-fix workouts, specialized equipment, and dietary supplement claims proliferate the media. Very few, if any, of these techniques and gadgets have any impact on preventing or delaying the onset of these disease states. Jeanne reiterates this point throughout her treatise. Why fall victim to anything more than—just move and move often—every day!!

---Ralph La Forge, MSc
   Clinical Lipid Specialist
   Clinical Exercise Physiologist
   Duke University - Endocrine Division
   Durham, NC

INTRODUCTION

What is quackery? Quackery is a false or misleading claim. A claim is a statement that something is true. Fitness companies often fall into the category of quackery, while trying to find and use that "key" word or phrase to reel in a customer. Americans spend millions of dollars each year believing and buying into luring claims, thereby becoming suckers.

So much quackery exists in this country, even in just the health and fitness industry, that it would be a lifetime project for me to write about it all. Therefore, in this book, I will only cover claims regarding weight loss/gain, muscle toning, flexibility, exercise technique, athletic performance, energy, "sound" nutrition, and fitness professionals.

The chapters are categories of fitness products and services: exercise equipment, nutrition, media, fitness "professionals," surgery and drugs, and miscellaneous. Also, there exists a chapter on exercise and nutrition myths. Although it is easy for you to leaf through this book to find the product or service that you are considering as an investment, I prefer that you read this book from cover to cover. It contains a lot of information about fitness that might not be repeated among products. Please take the time to learn.

An unlisted product or service is not necessarily free of quackery. It simply did not make my lists.

This book was originally written in 1997, but was not published until 2016. Although some of the products that were available in 1997 were not on the market at the time of printing, they remained in this book as a learning tool. Besides, as you'll find, through the years the product names change, but the quackery remains the same.

One reason why it took so long for me to publish this book is because of all the negative comments I made about a lot of people, services, and products. Not even my lawyer could tell me how to write it differently to prevent a lawsuit. So, I decided to change the names and add satire. In a way, it doesn't matter what the names are, because misleading claims are recycled. The bottom line for me is that you get my point. The bottom line for you is that you learn to recognize and avoid quackery in order to protect your health and wealth.

Consult your physician before starting an exercise conditioning program. The risks of exercising may include disorders of heartbeats, abnormal blood pressure response, and, very rarely, a heart attack. Consult a registered dietitian if you have special dietary needs.

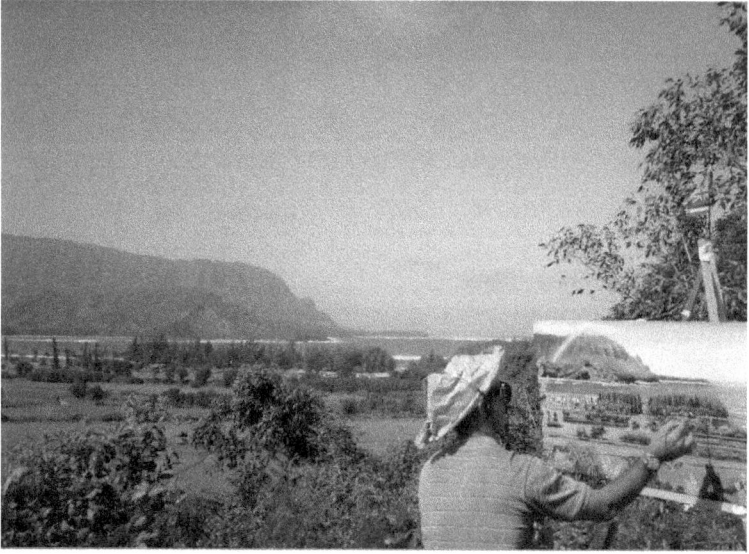

It's OK for artists to tweak the truth.

Hanalei Bay, Kauai, Hawaii

CHAPTER 1

EXERCISE EQUIPMENT

Along with the fitness craze comes exercise equipment/gadgets, many of those claiming to be "just what you need." Some are truly effective and well-made, but the manufacturers' claims are often invalid—quackery. They might promise you quick results! easy movements! little work! little time commitment! The better it sounds, the more likely it is quackery. Exercise requires a lifelong commitment of a daily routine with a lot of effort.

Another problem associated with the equipment includes improper demonstrations. Pictures or videos of models using a product often demonstrate either bad form or a contraindicated (known to be risky) movement. Always consult a qualified personal fitness trainer before using any exercise equipment.

The exercise products listed below are ones that I saw advertised in a variety of media sources. The manufacturers sent me information upon my request. Some of the information I requested was never sent to me, so it did not make my list. Also, some of the products I researched did not have quackery and therefore did not make my list, either. Other products not on my list may be ones that I have never heard of or came out after publication. Some companies may have cleaned up their acts before publication; their past misguidance will serve as an effective teaching tool, anyway.

I put an asterisk after a brand name I changed for my protection. The fictitious name doesn't necessarily have anything to do with the product; it's just designed to make you laugh.

Electro-Muscular Stimulation

Electro-Muscular Stimulation (EMS) is a non-invasive procedure that causes targeted muscles to contract and relax. Signals are sent via electrodes in the form of conductive rubber pads, mimicking brain impulses that would be present during exercise.

Before EMS was marketed toward lazy Americans who would be willing to pay anything not to exercise, yet look toned, it was primarily used in the physical therapy setting. It assists in the healing process of injured muscles or tendons (connect muscles to bones), and helps prevent atrophy (muscle loss) in those who are too sick or injured to exercise. Even in the rehabilitation setting, exercise—especially strength training—is done in conjunction with EMS as much as possible. You will not find a reputable physical therapist who advocates replacing strength training exercises with EMS. There are too many benefits of exercise, besides toning, that EMS cannot achieve.

In a setting where a company is providing EMS sessions in place of exercise, the sessions last about one hour. Below are some claims (quackery remember), that were highlighted in an EMS brochure:

". . . an easier and safer alternative means of physical fitness . . . [for] those with limited time for physical conditioning programs." Strength training sessions can be as short as 30 minutes to attain results, which is half as long as some EMS sessions. By the way, you will need to have EMS for the rest of your life if you want to maintain the muscle tone that you have developed, if any. Once you stop the procedure, your muscles will return to the state they were before you started, assuming you are still not exercising.

Supposedly, cardiovascular exercise and proper eating habits are encouraged complements to EMS, but I doubt that many EMS users would comply. If I were lazy enough to avoid strength training, why would I bother with the other two? Anyway, the brochure said that *cardiovascular exercise and good nutrition,* not EMS, help decrease fat stores, but then I read "EMS can get rid of cellulite caused by poor muscle tone and poor circulation." So, which is it? It is definitely cardiovascular exercise and good nutrition.

"Often times routine exercises become a burden . . ." No reputable health professional would tell people that exercise is a burden or concur with a client who comments as such. Exercise is a critical part of maintaining an independent, healthy lifestyle. If exercise is a burden, then so is wellness.

"EMS . . . will provide results much quicker than using traditional exercise programs." Faster is not better. The body needs to shift toward its healthier state slowly or else it will go into conservation mode. For example, when one loses weight quickly, from any means, the body responds by reducing its metabolism (rate at which Calories are burned). It wants to conserve energy so that it can have enough to sustain itself. Keep in mind that changes need to occur slowly to achieve success. Patience is a key factor in weight loss.

What can strength training exercises offer you that EMS cannot? Just to name a few: improve posture, balance, anxiety level, joint flexibility, and work productivity.

In conclusion, don't waste your time in an EMS session unless it is in conjunction with physical therapy.

Leg Slender*

Leg Slender, designed for one to sit and push independently moving foot pedals, includes handles that can be pushed and pulled. The hydraulic machine apparently gives one a cardiovascular and strength training workout concurrently.

First of all, this is a product endorsed by actress Slim-da Evans*. I am sure that she is a wonderful person. I just do not want you to choose a product, because you recognize a pretty face on the box (unless it's mine). Choose one because a qualified professional endorses it, as with Covert Bailey and the HealthRider.

Secondly, when I called the company that sold Leg Slender, a representative advised me of some interesting information. He said just "jump right out of bed and start exercising." Scientific reports have suggested that people with heart problems should not exercise first thing in the morning due to it being a shock to the body. Going from such a restful state to a high level of activity puts too much stress on the heart.

When is the best time of day to exercise?
The best time is when you will do it.

The claim is faulty, because it mandates when to exercise. No one can tell people when to exercise, since it is difficult enough just to get them to do it. The more limitations that are put on the public, the less likely they are to "bother" with working out. I agree that you should not just jump right out of bed and start exercising, because you need to warm the muscles first (by walking around, e.g.). Additionally, breakfast is a requirement for everyone, whether or not they exercise in the morning. It fuels the body, which fasted for several hours, and provides energy for the morning and exercise. Exercising on an empty stomach may cause a hypoglycemic (low blood sugar) reaction, resulting in nausea, dizziness, and fainting.

As for people with heart problems, if they want to exercise in the morning, they can do so after being awake for a little while. A lot of people know that if they do not workout before their day starts, they will not do it at all. Anyone, especially with a heart condition, should exercise.

Since a warm-up is required before starting strength training, stretching, or moderate- to high-intensity cardiovascular exercise, a morning exerciser should do a longer than normal (five minutes minimum) warm-up.

Now, back to Leg Slender: ". . . get the best results in the morning," the representative told me. Well, the results will not be any different in the morning than it will in the afternoon or evening. ". . . spike[s] metabolism in the morning and then it slowly declines throughout the day." That is true, but exercising every day (at any hour), your metabolism will stay at a relatively higher, consistent level than if no exercise had been done at all.

Onto the brochures I received. One had testimonials from four different people. Testimonials are supportive quotations from people who have used a product or service. I do not believe in using these, because they suggest that others will benefit the same way. Notice. "When I'm using the [Leg Slender] I can see that my legs, thighs and quads are tightening and toning. You can tell where it's working," says one customer. What if you are so fat that you cannot see those muscles contracting? Will you discontinue using the product and stop exercising? Many overweight people's muscles benefit from exercising, but cannot be noticed, due to the thick fat layer. If you adhere to an exercise program long enough to reduce the fat, though, the tonicity will show.

"I was impressed by what a great workout it was. Within 5 minutes, my heart rate was up," explains another customer. Any physical activity will increase your heart rate—it does not take a special machine. By the way, exercise causes an immediate heart rate response—you do not have to wait five minutes.

"In just 3-1/2 weeks, I lost 8 1/2 pounds* and 6 inches," boasts a customer. As the asterisk (*) explains, results vary. That is a very important point to clarify. Were the six inches in one place or two in each the chest, waist, and hips, for example? I wouldn't want inches lost in my chest; it's already small enough. Was the weight lost just fat or muscle, too? What else was done in the 3 1/2 weeks? This testimonial is deceiving, because you do not know what else was done. Also, the brochure suggests fast results. Remember that faster is not better—one kilogram or 2.2 pounds is the safe weight limit to lose in one week.

"You see almost instant results! [Leg Slender] really made a change in my workout program. I lost a total of 8* pounds!" "Almost" instant results? No exercise provides instant results. It can take six to eight weeks, after the onset of an exercise conditioning program, for muscle growth to occur. The body needs constant, consistent stressing (positive), before it will change. Also, altering the workout program is required to get off of a plateau and improve. Strength training routines should be changed every three months to keep the muscles and the mind stimulated. A cardiovascular exercise routine should be changed regularly, also, to continue challenging the body.

Another brochure states that you will ". . . melt away fat . . ." Fat does not melt away. It is not as though your body heat melts fat like stove heat melts butter. During exercise, fat is used as a fuel, which means that its chemical structure is broken down via enzymes, resulting in byproducts such as ATP (adenosine triphosphate—energy), heat, and water.

". . . without undue stress to knees." If you do it wrong, it will hurt your knees. Make sure that your knees do not bend more than a 90-degree angle *or* straighten to the point of being locked. You do need to straighten them all the way, stopping just before they lock.

This machine combines "muscle strengthening and aerobic conditioning." I can understand how it could strengthen your lower body, but Leg Slender should not replace strength training per se, i.e. weight lifting. This product should be thought of as cardiovascular exercise, not strength training. No such equipment can replace strength training. Only actual strength training exercises can count as strength training.

"We developed . . . especially for women." Men cannot use it?

Wow! Read what fine print I just read: "Models portraying dramatized testimonials." No!!?? Really!!?? Wait. You mean what was written was not really true and did not happen? Isn't that lying? Hmm. I have read a lot of quackery, but I have never seen it admitted before.

The videotape I received was similar to an infomercial, in that it had more testimonials. Slim-da Evans once said, "I guarantee you," when talking about results. No reputable fitness professional would ever guarantee results, because every body responds differently to exercise. When my personal training clients asked me if I guaranteed results, I responded, "Do you guarantee that you'll do everything that I suggest?" You can imagine that I heard crickets after that question. Also the video suggested to do 20-30 minutes for optimal results, but failed to say that some people need to start off doing only five minutes and that some need to work up to doing two hours worth to attain a healthy percentage of fat. Lastly, something funny I saw was a dumbbell rack next to one person who was on the machine. Why would she need weights if she has Leg Slender? Remember that they claim that their machine is the only thing that you will ever need for exercise?

Leg Slender costs "only" $399.95. Hmm. Walking costs nothing . . . well, you need a good pair of walking shoes . . . and you will attain the same results.

Although I have not tried this machine, it does not look like a bad one. I just do not want you to buy it, because of being reeled in from the misleading claims, or have false hopes. If you do own it, use a relaxed grip on the handles, since having clenched hands can increase your blood pressure more than it normally would during exercise. Make sure that your elbows do not straighten to the point of being locked.

Soft Walker*

Soft Walker, a foldaway treadmill, has a cushioned belt with "energy-absorbing material."

The brochure I received did not have much quackery in it, except hand weights are included in the package that comes with the treadmill. During cardiovascular exercise, such as walking or running, you should not wear ankle weights, wrist weights, or hold dumbbells, because it puts excessive stress on the joints and alters gait (manner of walking).

Often, weights are a suggested complement to tone and strengthen muscles and increase heart rate. Tone and strengthen muscles separately. Increase your heart rate by moving faster on the treadmill or increasing the grade.

This treadmill, overall, looks like a pretty good one.

Ego Flex*

If you have ever watched any television at all, then you are familiar with the Ego Flex machine. Does a guy or girl with a beautiful body ring a bell? It seems as though this company pioneered infomercials, or at least for exercise equipment. Ego Flex, designed for home use, provides a means for performing several strength training exercises on one machine. The machine includes attachable rubber bands and a bar on which plates can be added.

After my inquiry, I received a pamphlet and videotape. The brochure states that "[Ego Flex] delivers results identical to freeweights . . ." Actually, only free weights (e.g., dumbbells, barbells, and ankle weights) can deliver results identical to free weights, since they are exactly how they sound—free. Since they are not attached to any stationary object while you are using them, they require much more balance and coordination than machines. Although I like free weights a lot, machines are nice, too. I am just illustrating that there exist benefits of free weights over machines.

I did not like that on one page of the brochure, the phone number to call to place an order was stamped right on a girl's chest. No, you do not have to see this author's name—mine—to know that I am female. OK. So, I do not mind seeing the phone number placed on the guy's waistline on the next page. Here we go again. Now I see on yet another page the phone number printed right below a woman's symphisis pubis (where the two pelvic bones join—i.e., the crotch). All three placements are a bit much.

Of course testimonials exist, too, by people who say that they have lost weight by using the machine. They neglect to say that they (probably) were eating better and doing cardiovascular exercise, too. All four aspects—healthy eating, cardiovascular exercise, strength training, and stretching—are necessary for a well-rounded weight loss program.

"Aerobic-only exercises like treadmills . . . do not build any muscle." That is true to a certain extent. If a non-exerciser starts walking, he will add some muscle and get a little stronger in the legs, but will not achieve his potential muscle development without strength training.

"The most effective way to burn fat is to lift weights." Strength training raises your metabolism by building muscle, which can help to burn fat, but cardiovascular exercise actually uses fat as a fuel. This is one reason why both are necessary to do. "I lost three inches in my waist (and I was no longer doing any aerobic exercise)," states a customer. Ego Flex insinuates that aerobic exercise is not necessary, but it is! Aerobic exercise offers many benefits that strength training alone does not, such as decreasing resting heart rate, lowering cholesterol, and increasing maximum heart rate and cardiac output.

Ego Flex actually increases "your aerobic capacity because you have more working muscles taking in oxygen!" Well, maybe a little. Using Ego Flex requires the body's anaerobic (burning Calories without oxygen) system to work, whereas aerobic exercise uses the aerobic system. Maximum aerobic capacity (VO_2 max) is measured in milliliters of oxygen per kilogram of body weight per minute (ml/kg/min). In other words, it is the greatest amount of oxygen your body can utilize in order to burn Calories. Since oxygen is not needed during *anaerobic* exercise, VO_2 max is increased, primarily, by taxing the body *aerobically*.

You should not copy the exercise form of two of the pictured exercisers. One is doing a shoulder press (in a seated position, pushing bar above head) with extended wrists (hands bent back), which puts a tremendous amount of stress on those joints. Also, there is no means for back support at all. Another person, doing a similar exercise with wrists extended, too, has her feet tucked backward. When seated, the ankles need to be directly under the knees to place the back in its neutral position, or else there will be negative stress on the back. Lastly, all of the abdominal exercises pictured in another Ego Flex brochure are dangerous for the back. Do not perform these!

In the larger pamphlet, two smaller handouts were included to promote their free weights and Sock-it* (sounds like another ego maneuver—a pair of socks in a man's drawers) machine. Why do they offer free weights if the Ego Flex is supposed to be all that one needs? Anyway, do not follow the form or exercise suggestions in the dumbbell brochure—many are wrong. As for Sock-it, a machine that simulates squats and lunges, do not follow these pictured exercises, either. As *always*, consult a reputable personal fitness trainer, first. See Chapter 4 for the definition of reputable.

The video I was sent included people demonstrating exercises on the Ego Flex. In each example, the person was doing at least one thing wrong. Form and safety are emphasized, but they obviously do not know what proper form is. This is especially true with the abdominal exercises, as I mentioned earlier. Plus, the voice on the video added that one could work the "lower and upper abs." This suggests that you can isolate the upper and lower parts of the rectus abdominis (the six-pack) muscle, which travels vertically down the front of the abdomen. Different parts of certain muscles can be isolated, but not this one. If the upper part is going to contract, then the whole length will. Yet, you might not feel much in the lower part, because that is where the muscle "thins out" and becomes tendon.

This machine does not look as versatile as it is advertised. It offers no back support for the seated exercises or enough adjustments to accommodate different-size people, correctly. Use your money elsewhere.

Ab Jerk*

Ab Jerk is a device for doing crunches. It is a board with hinges and handles, which supposedly allows you to perform crunches safely.

"I've gone down 4 sizes. I can now fit into my old jeans. My progress has been right in my range of goals and beyond!" exclaims the owner. Well, you know what I think about testimonials. What else did he do, if anything, besides Ab Jerk? If he achieved those results, does it mean that you will, too? By 4 sizes does he mean that he went from drinking a huge to a small container of cola daily? How strange to make a testimonial about one's own product or service. *Jeanne is the best writer ever and she always knows how to make me laugh* (even that made me laugh)!

"Trimmer, tighter abs and a slimmer waistline can be yours in just 5 minutes every other day!" That is all? So, they are saying this machine is all one has to use and for only 5 minutes every other day? Oh. As I continue reading, they imply that that statement was quackery. "Combined with a healthy diet and aerobic exercise, [Ab Jerk] can help you achieve . . ."

Also, with this product you can work your "lower abs." Remember that there is no such thing.

Save your money. Do not buy this product or any other that is supposed to help you do crunches properly. The floor and a little instruction is all you need.

Norse Skier*

Norse Skier, a cross-country ski machine, simulates this movement well. Cross-country skiing provides an excellent cardiovascular workout. "You'll burn 20% more calories on a [Norse Skier] than working out on an ordinary treadmill* (*University of Wisconsin research, LaCrosse, 1994)." You will not burn a lot of Calories if you do not use your skier. No kidding, right? It does not matter what great exercise a movement or machine offers if you do not use it.

When choosing a mode for cardiovascular exercise, you need to consider what you like, how much you want to spend (if anything), how coordinated you are, where you want to exercise, and whether or not you want to learn something new. If you have never cross-country skied, and do not care to learn, you should not buy a skier just because it is great exercise. You need to choose an exercise mode to which you will commit. If you like biking and are having second thoughts about doing it, because you heard that stair climbing is better for you, then ignore the claim. Bike. Choose what you like, since you will probably commit to it.

One- and half-pound grips are available accessories for the skier. Do not bother. It is like wearing wrist weights while walking—too much stress on the joints.

Lastly, the advertisement shows a girl twisting to look over her left shoulder, while on the skier. Do not twist, while skiing, because it negatively stresses your back.

Stroll Fit*

Stroll Fit looks like a combination of a treadmill and a cross-country ski machine. It has a belt on which one can walk and handles that can be pushed and pulled.

"Because [Stroll Fit] works both your lower and upper body, you can tone up your body and enjoy improved cardiovascular fitness at the same time." That may be so, but remember that strength training still needs to be done separately.

"For weight loss, work out for 30 minutes a day 3-4 times per week." For weight loss, work out for two hours six days a week. What if the advertisement said that? Would people buy the machine? Of course not. That advice would scare people away. Most people, especially those who do not like exercising, want fast results with little time commitment. But, did I state something realistic? Yes. Of course one would not start an exercise program, doing two hours six days a week, but some people need to work up to that volume to achieve a healthy percentage of body fat. It is alright if you do not commit a lot of time, now, for exercising, but eventually you might need to exercise two hours per day.

Stroll Fit also offers weighted workout gloves to use with this product. Do not buy these; they are just as harmful as using wrist weights while aerobically exercising.

Stroll Fit looks like a safe product, otherwise.

Roman Chair

A roman chair is a stand with an elevated, horizontal pad on which your pelvis goes (face up or down) and elevated padded rollers under which your feet go. Picture yourself on this stand horizontally (parallel to the floor) face up or down, moving your torso toward and away from the floor.

"Build tight abs and a strong back. Work your upper and lower abs, increase flexibility, and strengthen your back and abdominals safely and efficiently for superior results," one brand claims. No, no, no, no, no. You already know what I think about the term "lower abs." This chair should absolutely not be used for performing abdominal exercises, because it puts tremendous strain on the lower back, even if done carefully. As for lower back exercises, you would need to use great caution and a smart personal trainer, while on this chair. Avoid this chair if you have back or neck problems, have been exercising for fewer than six months, and have high blood pressure. Very rarely do I see anyone use this chair properly. There are many safe floor exercises for the lower back.

Ego Stand*

These types of stands include an elevated vertical pad, against which your back goes, and arm rests with handles. Using a step, you prop yourself up with your back against the pad and hold yourself up with your arms, feet dangling.

The idea is to raise and lower your legs, bending at the hip, knees straight or bent.

Must I use more no's? "Target all your abdominal muscle groups for excellent toning, trimming and conditioning . . . without undue stress on your lower back . . . to work your obliques [a pair of muscles on either side of your abdomen—used in twisting and bending], upper and lower abs for a great workout." Rarely have I seen people work their abdominal muscles on this stand, because doing so is a very difficult exercise. How this stand is advertised to be used puts a lot of compression force on the spine and does not activate the abdominal muscles, except in an isometric contraction. The stand offers a means for working the hips, only. Save your money. Choose safe floor exercises for the abdomen.

Flab Board*

These boards sit at a 45-degree angle (head toward floor), with rollers at one end to which your legs attach. The board is designed for performing sit-ups, which are contraindicated—known to be risky—at any angle.

Rower

Rowing machines provide a great cardiovascular workout. In one ad the model leans back at the end of the pulling motion. Although this rowing motion is common, I teach people to keep their backs straight the whole time. For most people, leaning back will put a negative stress on the lower back, resulting in back aches and strained lower back muscles. Be careful.

Norse Rider*

Norse Rider has a seat and a backrest, foot pedals to push, and bars in front for the exerciser to push and pull.

Norse Rider appears to be a nice piece of equipment that would offer an effective cardiovascular workout, but make sure that you do not extend your wrists like the girl in the ad does. Whenever you hold handles or free weights, *always* keep your wrists straight—as though you have a splint going across the front and back of your wrist so that they cannot be moved. When your palms have pressure against them and your hands are bent back (especially) or forward, it puts tremendous stress on the wrists. You can develop carpal tunnel syndrome from exercising improperly.

Carpal tunnel syndrome, often caused by repetitive movements, occurs in the wrist where a nerve passes through an opening in the wrist where the carpal bones are. Repetitive movements with the wrist in extension cause one or more tendons to inflame and press against the nerve, resulting in hand tingling and pain.

Strength training wrists and forearms is an exception when it is acceptable (and necessary) to bend your wrists, which is safe to do. Imagine holding a dumbbell in one hand; keeping that forearm parallel to the floor, move your fist up and down.

Norse Rider provides a safe, no-impact exercise that works your lower and upper body.

Circuit Training Bike*

Circuit Training Bike (CTB) looks like a stationary bicycle with handlebars that are multi-functional.

CTB "combines aerobics, complete muscle conditioning and total body stretching in ONE compact fitness machine!" "Six fast muscle toning exercises work all your major muscle groups for a firm, toned body . . ." Six are not only too few for a complete workout, but also too few to provide variety when it comes time to changing the strength training routine. A program of nine exercises is the minimum I prescribe to target all of the major muscle groups, including isolating the triceps and biceps (back and front of upper arm, respectively) and lower back. On the CTB you cannot do those. As for other routines, it is necessary to change your workout every three months to keep the muscles and the mind stimulated. You should have a means of doing different exercises when the time comes to change your program.

In the ad, the girl on the CTB has her wrists extended, which you now know is bad. Also, the machine does not have back support for doing the shoulder press exercise. Most people would need the support to avoid injuring the lower back.

Use this machine for cardiovascular exercise, only.

Fitness Jerks*

"The personal trainer for everybody." Oh, no! Do not put me out of business! "The [Fitness Jerks] is designed by . . . exercise physiologists to help you achieve your fitness goals through an easy step-by-step process. Simply watch the self-assessment video, add up your score and follow the video program designed for your fitness level." Included are ". . . 5 exercise videos with multiple exercise programs." So, they are already programmed? Yes! Then, it cannot be *personalized*. Gotcha! If the tape has already been made, then your fitness goals and medical background were not taken into consideration. *That* is what a personal trainer's role is: to learn what he can about the client, then prescribe a workout.

The price of this program could get you at least two sessions with a qualified personal trainer. Hire one, instead.

Weight Bar

This bar is just what it sounds like—a bar.

The "bodysculpting" bar, used to perform exercises, only adjusts to eight pounds, which most people—even unfit—would grow out of quickly. In order to show muscle improvement, you need to challenge the muscles, always, which means increasing the resistance as the muscles become stronger. Eight pounds does not allow you to continue increasing the resistance for very long.

Fat Flyer*

Fat Flyer has free-flowing pedals, on which you stand, and bars to move back and forth. The movement looks like cross-country skiing, but the pedals are in the air.

"Don't walk, run, ski or ride!" Because, they want you to spend lots of money on yet another gizmo. Rest assured that walking, running, skiing, and riding are still excellent cardiovascular exercise modes.

It gives you a "complete workout in just 20 minutes." Well, some people won't last more than five, while others will need to work up to doing more than one hour. No set time exists that people need to spend to achieve their fitness goals—everyone is unique.

". . . get a sexier . . . body . . ." Who does not want to look and feel sexy? Let us not forget the most important reason why we need exercise: to promote a long, healthy, independent lifestyle. Also, how do you perceive sexy? Is it someone you saw in a magazine, or how you looked a few years ago, for example? Be realistic and set realistic goals.

A machine can help you achieve your potential "beauty," but not achieve another person's body.

Fat Flyer might be fun to use, but make sure that you keep your tummy and chest against the pads, so that you do not hurt your back.

PowerBlock

PowerBlock, an adjustable dumbbell made by IntellBell, uses valid claims in its advertising, but the promotional tape needs a lot of work. There was not any verbal quackery in the tape, but many of the exercises were demonstrated improperly. If you ever watch the tape in consideration of buying the product, which is well made, keep in mind that many of the exercises are done wrong. Be sure to consult a qualified trainer if you invest in these weights. Do not follow the videotape.

Bowflex

Bowflex, a universal-type strength training machine, has approximately 10 rods used for resistance. As with many other similar machines, it includes a bench, cables, and handles.

I received brochures and videotape, describing the Bowflex and what exercises it allows you to execute. Actually, I was pretty impressed with the machine. It looks quite versatile, convenient to store, and easy to switch from one exercise to another.

Some quackery in the enclosed information did exist, though. ". . . strength training work[s] better than aerobics for getting fit and losing fat." *Both* aerobics and strength training are very important for getting fit and losing fat. One is not more important than the other is. As for losing fat, aerobics helps to burn the fat directly—during exercise—while strength training builds muscle, which increases the metabolism and enhances fat burning around the clock.

"We guarantee results because we want you to try Bowflex." EXACTLY! These companies are "guaranteeing" results in order to get you to buy the equipment. I have never guaranteed results to any of my clients, because I do not know exactly how their body will respond to exercise or how much they will eventually need to reach their goals. I asked my mentor, a few years ago, what my answer should be when someone asks me if I guarantee results. He replied, "Ask them, 'do you guarantee that you'll do what I say?'"

Side note: Do not hire a trainer unless you will do everything he suggests. Do not waste your time and money or his time. If you have a trainer, already, and do not trust everything he says, then it is time to hire a different one.

There were plenty of testimonials, of course, which I had the opportunity to hear and read. "I lost over 60 pounds of fat and 12 inches off my waist with Bowflex!" How long did it take? How drastically was the diet changed? What other exercises, if any, were performed? Does that mean everyone would achieve these same results? No.

"Absolute best way to reshape your body." There exists no best way to "reshape your body" or one best exercise. Well, OK. One exception:

The best exercise is that which is done.

Lastly, most of the exercises I saw demonstrated on the video were great examples with proper form, except for four—three abdominal movements and one shoulder movement. Consult a trainer, anyway, before using this equipment to learn which routine works best for you.

Flab Blaster*

You must remember this piece of equipment . . . endorsed by Cezanne Summers*. It has two royal blue horseshoe-shaped pads connected by a red hinge. You are supposed to put the device between your legs and squeeze the pads toward each other for great-looking thighs.

It takes a lot more than a Flab Blaster to achieve great-looking thighs. First, there are many other muscles that give the thighs their shape. This device only works about one fourth of the thigh muscles. Second, people need to exercise aerobically to lose some fat over the muscles, so that their definition can be seen. Lastly, proper nutrition is a must. You will not keep the fat off, after exercising, if you continue to consume more Calories than you are burning. Oh. Having the genetic disposition toward obtaining your definition of "great-looking thighs" helps, too.

Weight Vest

This vest can be worn during a workout or just . . . around. It can hold up to ten pounds to help you burn more Calories during your workout. Apparently a 130-pound woman will burn 25 more Calories in one hour of walking with the vest than without the vest.

So, do *you* need this vest? Probably not. You can burn more than 25 extra Calories by simply increasing your pace and variable terrain training—going up and down hills.

Pear Body*

Pear Body sells home strength training equipment, which include weight stacks. The universal-type machines are designed to perform several different exercises on it. I like this equipment a lot and use it with some of my clients.

There were not any false claims in the brochures, regarding what the equipment could do for you, but there were improperly-performed exercises. One shoulder exercise could injure the shoulders. There is a safer way to do it, but that is what you would need to learn from a trainer.

Why can't you learn exercises from these equipment manufacturers? You should be able to, but I have seen so many brochures that include contraindicated exercises and ones that are done wrong. So, why don't they demonstrate the proper movements? I do not know. I guess they are not using the proper experts, such as myself, who know biomechanics. Update: money. After I wrote the first version of this book, many exercise equipment manufacturers frankly told me that they don't care that models are demonstrating the equipment wrong. "As long as we're making money, we're happy."

Anyway, I like and recommend Pear Body. Consult a personal trainer, before using it, to learn *your* ideal workout.

Yuck-on*

Yuck-on sells home and gym fitness equipment, which looks well made. Although in their brochure, too, the model performs some exercises with her wrists extended (ouch!) and one that is contraindicated—bad for the back, in this case.

Flab Isolator*

Tiny Vittles*, a personal fitness trainer, endorses the Flab Isolator, another device used for crunches. It "targets upper and lower abdominals." Remember that there is no such thing as upper and lower abdominals. It "locks your legs and hips in place." You do not need to have your legs and hips locked in place if you are performing crunches properly. "As far as I'm concerned, you will never need another abdominal product," Tiny claims. As far as *I'm* concerned, you do not need *any* abdominal product. I have yet to find anyone who cannot perform abdominal exercises properly, without a device, and I have worked with a lot of unconditioned people.

Some abdominal devices provide head and neck support, but so does a towel. Try putting a kitchen towel behind your neck with the ends pointing in the direction of your face. Grab onto the left side with your right hand and the right side with your left hand. Your arms will cross, but the towel will not, because you do not want to put pressure on your carotid (neck) arteries. Relax your head in the towel and keep your hands a bit relaxed—no death grip. Use your abdominal muscle to pull you up, while your head is relaxed and just along for the ride. Use your hands to hold your head and towel only, not to pull you up.

Health for Now*

Health for Now sells many types of exercise and nutritional products. One supplement they offer contains creatine "for increased anaerobic power, higher caloric expenditure, and faster recovery." See chapter 2 for information on creatine. No pill or powder will give you great abs.

"When abs are on the agenda, no health club or home gym should be without these big, colorful charts." The wall chart with suggested abdominal exercises has three examples of improperly performed movements. Actually, two or three others are contraindicated abdominal exercises, since they put tremendous pressure on the back and neck. I could not quite read the fine print on the chart, but I bet that it was made in the '80s.

The rest of Health For Now's claims appear reasonable. I like the rest of the products they offer, most of which are marketed to bodybuilders. Other products include forearm strengtheners, books, videotapes, and workout gloves.

Facial Devices

Devices used to build facial muscles appeared on the market long ago. The manufacturers claim the devices help hold up sagging faces by building facial muscles. But the UC Berkeley Wellness Letter of February 1997 deems the devices ineffective, since sagging skin comes from sun exposure and genetics, not sagging muscles. I agree.

Fat Trainer*

Fat Trainer requires you to "grasp the front handlebars and rock slowly backwards in the pivoting seat, extending tight muscles. An included workout video demonstrates eight stretches: "Lower back. Hamstring (back of thigh). Gluteal, hip. Hip, leg, back. Inner thigh, groin. Upper back. Shoulders. Quadricep." That is nice, but stretching does not require a machine or special chair, since stretches can easily be performed on the floor or in a regular chair, if necessary. Also, remember to stretch the rest of the upper body, neck, and torso sides (obliques).

Leg Builder*

Leg Builder, primarily designed for squatting, includes a rack that holds a harness. The harness sits on the rack, while you attach weight, and then sits on your shoulders while you perform an exercise.

"Squatting is the best exercise for developing the thighs and building lower body strength. But aside from the pain of holding the barbell on your shoulders, heavy squatting is hard on the knees and lower back and will enlarge the buttocks. Now it is possible to develop your legs without having to endure the discomfort of barbell squats." First of all, no "best exercise" exists. Second, heavy squatting does not hurt the knees and lower back, if performed correctly and progressed slowly. As a matter of fact, the demonstrator in the Leg Builder ad performs the squats improperly, such that a tremendous amount of negative stress is placed on the knees. When squatting, your rear should stick out, like you are about to sit in a chair. The knees should stay over the ankles with your thighs going no lower than parallel to the floor.

Even with proper form, I am not sure how useful the Leg Builder is. It might be uncomfortable to have the harness on your shoulders, when exercising correctly.

Before you buy exercise equipment . . . before you *research* exercise equipment, ask yourself these questions:

1. What types of cardiovascular exercise do I like doing?
2. What type of cardiovascular exercise am I most likely to do consistently?
3. Where will I exercise? (e.g., home, park, gym)
4. Realistically, will I use the product consistently long term?
5. Will I consult a trainer, after purchase, to learn how best to use the equipment?
6. Do I really need the equipment to achieve a healthy lifestyle?
7. How much am I willing to spend?
8. What mode of strength training do I like best? (e.g., bands, free weights, machines, water)
9. Do I have room in my home for the equipment?
10. Who else will use the equipment?
11. Do I want to learn something new?
12. Am I able to test the equipment, before I buy, to see if it fits (is adjustable for) me.

Shop around. Be skeptical of the sounds-too-good-to-be-true claims.

Lastly, buy a product because you hope that it will make you feel and look your best, rather than to look like the model demonstrating it.

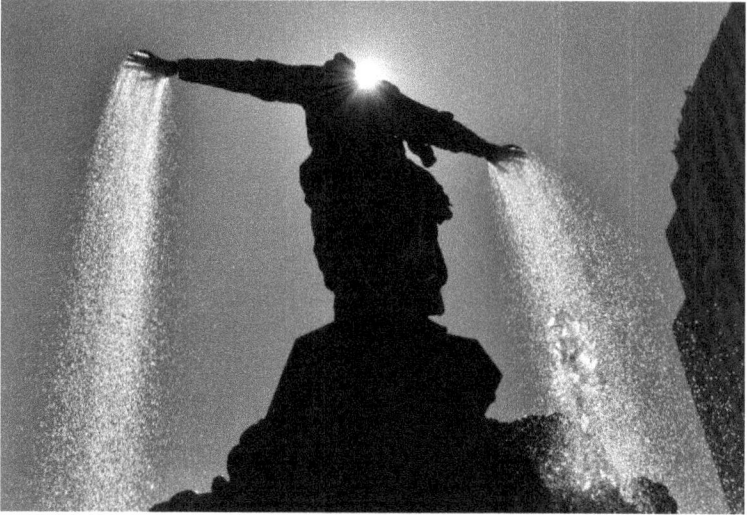

The Genius of Water, sculpture by Tyler Davidson

Cincinnati, Ohio

Water is the only true energy drink.

CHAPTER 2

NUTRITION

Anytime someone tells me one thing—one diet, one pill, one exercise—will help every problem from cancer to ingrown toenails, I am suspicious.

--Ann Grandjean, director of the Center for Human Nutrition in Omaha, Nebraska, on the promise of *The Zone* and other high-protein diets.

The following list of nutrition products include diets, supplements, sports drinks/bars, and ingredients that you might see in other products.

I put an asterisk after a brand name I changed for my protection. The fictitious name doesn't necessarily have anything to do with the product; it's just designed to make you laugh.

Therma Get-Its*

"Wanted: 96 PEOPLE. We will pay you to lose up to 30 pounds in the next 30 days. Offer expires" soon. Call 1-800-Quackery. This quick weight loss is not only unsafe but also unhealthy.

The safest amount to lose in one week is one kilogram or 2.2 pounds. The faster you lose weight, the more likely your metabolism will slam on the brakes to conserve energy, resulting in eminent weight gain at the cessation of the program.

I called the phone number and listened to a recording, after which time I requested information that I never received. Apparently Therma Get-Its is an herbal supplement that works "directly on metabolism, increase[s] your energy, and help[s] you not to crave sweets." Exercise works directly on metabolism, increases energy level, and helps suppress sweet craving, and it does not cost anything. Plus it has *many* other benefits. Judging by my experiences with nutritional counseling, most people's main diet problem includes overconsumption—not necessarily sweets or other *wrong* foods.

". . . lost over 43 pounds and 28 inches in 12 weeks." Does that mean you will? What else did the person do? Obese people do usually lose fat faster at the start of a weight loss program than thinner types who only need to lose a few pounds.

BE CAREFUL WITH HERBS! The FDA (Food and Drug Administration) has not tested every herb, yet. Be sure to know an herb's contraindications before taking it. Harmful herbs now circulate, so I would not even trust asking someone at a health food store, unless I am speaking to a registered dietitian or an eastern medicine expert, such as an acupuncturist. Health food store workers usually know only the claims that the manufacturers make.

Blind Vision Intentional*

This multi-level marketing company seems more interested in having you as a "member" (salesman) than as a product consumer.

They offer "nutritional" supplements of vitamins and minerals in the form of capsules and liquid, respectively. Following many of their claims, such as "Life-sustaining minerals are necessary for certain daily bodily functions," lies an asterisk (*). The fine print reads "These statements have not been evaluated by the Food and Drug Administration. This product is not intended to diagnose, treat, cure, or prevent any disease." In other words: *We are just blowing hot air to get you to buy our product; the FDA does not have time to get around to all of us—fortunately! We want you to think our product is the miracle drug. Whatever you do, do not read the fine print.*

"The importance of minerals in food is so new that the textbooks on nutritional dietetics contain very little about it." What books were *they* reading?

"Our physical well-being is more directly dependent upon the minerals we take into our systems than upon calories or vitamins, or upon the precise proportions of starch, protein or carbohydrates we consume." All of those aspects equally make up a balanced, healthy diet—one is not more important than the other.

The mineral product contains 900 mg/l of sodium and 720 mg/l of sulfur. That is a lot. We do not even need more than 500 mg/day of sodium, and it is obvious how salt-ridden the average American diet is, already. Experts approximate that we rack up 4000-5000 mg/day of sodium. It is recommended that we consume at most 2400 mg/day of sodium.

The vitamin product contains a "plant enzyme complex," which supposedly helps digest the fruit juice. Well, if you were eating fresh fruits, you would already be consuming enzymes . . . and fiber! Fiber, an important nutrient, is absent in supplements and juices. Eat the *whole* fruit or vegetable and you will get the *whole* benefit.

Among other products, this company sells pyruvate (also known as pyruvic acid), a naturally occurring substance resulting from carbohydrate metabolism. They "stimulate cellular mitochondria respiration, the cell's energy engine, and inhibit the body's deposition of fat." So does exercise—and it is free! The brochure cited a study where obese women went on a 1000-Calorie-per-day liquid diet in addition to taking pyruvate. Twelve hundred Calories should be the bare minimum that one consumes, since the body's metabolism slows down when it does not get enough food.

So, should you use this product? No. Should you use any vitamin or mineral supplement? Be careful. Some research has suggested yes, but it is still under speculation and without specific guidelines as to who should take how much of what. If you do take them, do not consume more than 100% of the RDA (recommended dietary allowance) for any given nutrient. Although minerals and the fat-soluble vitamins A, D, E, and K are easily stored, the water-soluble vitamins B and C also can be toxic in large amounts. One of the byproducts of vitamin C metabolism, oxalic acid, can build up in the kidneys and create kidney stones, whether or not one has the enzyme to break down this compound. An apparently healthy individual with a well-rounded diet does not need supplementation, but there are exceptions. One example includes people with osteoporosis, a bone disease, may need a large amount of calcium and vitamin D. Consult your doctor to determine if you have any medical reasons why you should consume an extra amount of any vitamin and mineral. He should have the last word, not a health food store clerk.

Norse Fat Pack*

"No time to eat right?" No time to eat correctly? No time to eat? The first question can be inferred two different ways. Regardless, this product insinuates that it is not only acceptable to eat poorly, but also not have time to eat. How is it that people don't have time to eat, but have time to overeat? Norse Fat Pack wants you to buy their supplements. Supplements are not a replacement for proper eating habits, as the word supplement is defined. Although, many people think that they can eat poorly, take a supplement, and still maintain their health. Vitamin/mineral manufacturers have wrongly influenced those people.

The nutrition system has ". . . a special metabolic conditioner to help your body burn fat . . . improve your lean body mass." Then why would anyone need one of this company's exercise machines? One would. There exists no magic pill for burning fat or gaining lean body mass, so do not believe any such claims. Exercise provides a means for fat burning and muscle gaining. The more fat you want to lose, the more you will need to workout, and the longer it will take you to reach your goals. Accept and comply with these words and you will achieve success through patience and hard work. Think about how many years it took you (those of you) to obtain your fat: years, eh? Losing excess fat will not be a short period, either.

This formula "is the perfect complement to your exercise routine." No. Proper eating habits offer the perfect complement to an exercise program.

Herbs-a-Lie*

Herbs-a-Lie, a pyramid company, sells products for weight management, skin care, hair, bath and body, and fragrances. Since my specialty lies in weight management, I will only critique those products.

Of course the brochure carries many testimonials and before and after photos of people who have lost weight from using the products. Do those testimonials guarantee that you will lose weight, too? No.

Almost every product touts a ridiculous claim like "weight-loss support in the evening," "produce a more desirable energy balance," and "naturally aids the body in absorbing less fat." One claim indirectly suggests that it is an appetite suppressant. Exercise can do all of those and it is free.

Instead of investing in pills, learn how to choose healthy foods, eat in moderation, and implement an exercise program. To be healthy, you need to create and maintain healthy habits for life. Taking expensive pills, which usually just make for expensive urine and stool, does not teach you how to live a healthy lifestyle. Most people who take supplements fool themselves by thinking that since they take certain pills, they can still continue their bad habits.

"[Money-U-Lose*] helps reduce the appearance of cellulite." Reduce the appearance of cellulite by reducing cellulite. Exercise!

Do not get sucked into using or selling Herbs-a-Lie. Besides, one who is without a nutrition degree should not be educating the public on nutritional supplements.

Vitamin B$_6$ (Pyridoxine)

Vitamin B$_6$ is "involved in more bodily functions than any other single nutrient, works against water retention, assists with the breakdown of fats . . . ," one medically-supervised weight loss program advertises. They prescribe this vitamin in supplement form for weight loss, when one should be able to attain enough from food. Vitamin B_6 can be found in meats, whole grains, legumes, and green leafy vegetables, among other foods. Some people do need supplements, but not for weight loss.

Vitamin B_{12} (Cyanocobalamin)

Vitamin B_{12} is "required for proper digestion, absorption of foods, synthesis of protein and metabolism of carbohydrates and fats . . ." True. We can attain B_{12} by eating fish and pork, eggs, cheese, and milk and milk products.

Soup diet

The soup diet's objectives are to change one's eating habits in a short period of time, to lose weight rapidly, and to prepare one for a low-carbohydrate diet. First of all, new habits take a while to create, and you should not expect overnight changes. Secondly, weight loss should be slow to be most effective, since the body will object to rapid losses and in turn decrease your metabolism. Thirdly, carbohydrates should comprise 55-58% of total daily Calories. People think that carbohydrates are bad, rationalizing that too much bread or pasta will make you fat. Too much of anything will make you fat! You need carbohydrates.

The diet plan, also known as Miracle Slop* or the Cabbage Soup Diet, touts "Lose 14-17 lbs. and feel like a million in only 7 days. One of the secrets of the effectiveness of the 7-day plan is that the foods eaten take more calories to burn than they give to the body in calorie value. So eat as much as you want." Losing that much weight in one week is far too much, unhealthy, unsafe, and can cause gallstones. It makes no sense that more Calories are burned in metabolizing the food than the amount of Calories the food provides. Your metabolism does increase after eating a meal, but not that much. Being able to eat as much as you want of any food does not teach you portion control and variety.

I have seen different recipes for this soup, which basically include one head of red cabbage, other vegetables (including canned), and onion soup mix. For the most part, it is healthy soup, actually, except for all of the salt. A lot of salt would come from the canned vegetables, the soup mix, and what the dieter is allowed to use.

The soup diet is unhealthy, because grains are not allowed until the seventh day, dairy products are only allowed on the fourth day, and meat only on the fifth and sixth days. We need to have all of the food groups *everyday*. Also, any diet that encourages *temporary* behavior should be avoided, but actually that is what diets are supposed to be—temporary. That is partly what makes them bad. Healthy eating habits should be permanent.

In this book, I do not aim to critique every diet or diet center that has ever existed. That would not only be a book in and of itself, but also a waste of time. I need you to accept that diets should be avoided, rapid weight loss can hurt you, and permanent healthy eating habits should be learned and adopted.

If you want a book that judges diets, read *Complete Food and Nutrition Guide* by Roberta Larson Duyff.

Lastly, I could cite research, which has proven that diets do not work, but all you have to do is ask yourself or someone you know, "Has any diet helped you lose fat, gain muscle, and maintain healthy body composition?" No's will be answered by 95% of the population.

Chromium Picolinate

"Chromium Picolinate! Reduce sugar cravings! Accelerate fat loss! Eat the foods you love! 100% safe and natural! Just a dollar a day!" A multi-level marketing company called Fat Intentional* makes these claims. Apparently, they only sell chromium—the main ingredient in their product Thermo Flab*, which also includes herbs.

Chromium, an essential mineral found in the blood, stimulates glucose metabolism for energy and the synthesis of fatty acids, cholesterol, and possibly protein. It "appears to increase the effectiveness of insulin and its ability to handle glucose, preventing hypoglycemia (too much insulin) or diabetes (too little insulin). The chromium-containing foods most biologically available to the body are brewer's yeast (the best), liver, beef, whole-wheat bread, beets and beet sugar molasses, and mushrooms" (Dunne 1990). In excess, chromium may aggravate diabetes.

"Many of the nation's most respected and widely-read newspapers have devoted articles to Chromium Picolinate, including *The Los Angeles Times, Washington Post, USA Today,* and *McCall's* just to name a few," Fat Intentional boasts. So? They are well-respected, but not medical journals. Newspapers and magazines will print anything that they think will get people's attention. Chromium picolinate is definitely one of those, since America is looking for a miracle drug.

I consider exercise the miracle elixir, because it is a miracle more people do not do it. It can help you lose weight *and* improve your sex life!

Melissa Hallmark, et al. (1996) studied the effects of chromium on body composition and strength. After a 12-week strength training program and chromium supplementation, the subjects showed no change in body fat or weight, skinfold thickness, and lean body mass. Although the subjects increased their strength, they also

41

increased their chromium excretion, which means that the extra mineral was not used. The placebo group also showed an increase in strength and no change in body weight.

Therefore, do not buy chromium picolinate.

Jenny Craig Weight Loss Center

I have never thought very highly about weight loss centers, because they usually sell people expensive diet food and promote fast weight loss. Also, they seem to be the epitome of quackery. The following excerpts come from an article I saw in the newspaper (Miller 1997), regarding misleading claims by Jenny Craig and other centers.

> La Jolla-based Jenny Craig Inc. has agreed to tone down some weight-loss claims as part of a settlement of deceptive-advertising charges, the Federal Trade Commission (FTC) announced yesterday.

> As part of the settlement, the company must warn consumers that weight loss is temporary for many dieters. Jenny Craig must also back any claims with scientific evidence and spell out all mandatory fees in its program.

> The settlement would end a lawsuit the FTC filed in September 1993 against Jenny Craig and Weight Watchers International Inc. The five FTC commissioners are now considering a settlement with Weight Watchers, commission spokeswoman Bonnie Jansen said. Three other diet organizations, Nutri/System Inc., Diet Center Inc. and Physician Weight Loss Centers Inc., settled similar FTC complaints in 1993, before lawsuits were filed.

In its suit, the government maintained that Jenny Craig advertising gave consumers unrealistic expectations about weight loss. The FTC also alleged that the company lacked the evidence to back contentions that customers would be able to dramatically lose weight and keep it off for a long time. There were further concerns about pricing claims and fears that potential health concerns were not adequately explained.

The settlement also requires that consumer testimonials be representative of what customers in general tend to achieve, unless, the government said, the advertisement "clearly and prominently discloses either the generally expected results or a statement such as: 'This result is not typical. You may be less successful.'"

The FTC said only 5 percent of the 50 million Americans who go on diets annually keep off the weight they lose. About 8 million of these are enrolled in a "structured weight-loss program," the government said.

This lawsuit demonstrates the unveiling of weight loss centers' façade which, for so many years, disguised the truth about dieting.

Juicing

Juicing, a process involving putting fruits and/or vegetables into a machine to liquefy them, became very popular many years ago. Juicing machine manufacturers promoted their products as a tasty means to consume a large volume of produce at once.

Juicing is a great way to get people to eat more produce, but it is very time consuming. I have seen even the most fanatic juicers get burned out because of the time commitment. The produce must be cleaned and put through the machine, and then the machine must be cleaned.

Also, a lot of nutrients are lost, especially fiber, because the skin or pulp of the fruits and vegetables are left behind. Most people throw out this important part, but the people who find some use for it benefit the most.

Lastly, it is better to consume fruits and vegetables throughout the day, than all in one sitting, to ensure absorption and usage of nutrients and to provide the body with an ongoing supply. For example, the body can only use half of a 1000 mg dose of calcium and the rest is excreted in urine. Therefore, two separate 500 mg servings are better.

Wheat Grass Juice

We are not cows . . .

OK, I will not just leave it at that, although I want to. Wheat grass juice is just like it sounds—liquefied lawn. You would most likely find it sold at juicing establishments. They grow the grass at the store and then put it in a juicer when ordered. It is supposedly packed with nutrients, but so is the produce at the supermarket.

Although I am trying to teach you how to save money, I dare you to try this juice. Warning: it is one of the nastiest things I have ever tasted. Do people drink it because it tastes good? I think not.

You do not need to drink this juice to be healthy.

I have to tell you that I will always remember a scene at a juicing business. A mother was holding a toddler and a cup of wheat grass juice that she offered the child. The child leaned back, put her hand up, and made a face that *I* would mimic when posed with the same offer. Smart kid.

Fasting

Fasting has been a weight-loss means even before diets per se were invented. Also, in certain religions, it is a means for "cleansing."

"'We don't need to fast to clean out our organs; they're constantly cleaning themselves,' says Dr. George Blackburn, an expert in nutritional medicine at Harvard Medical School" (deVries & Housh 1994).

Because it is too dangerous, there are few scientists who believe that fasting is an immune system stimulant. "When the body is deprived of food, it turns to its own resources for fuel—first to sugar molecules in the bloodstream, then, after about 24 hours, to stores of glycogen, or body fat. After a day or so more without food, when carbohydrates are depleted, the body starts to convert fat into chemical compounds called ketones. But when ketones accumulate in the kidneys, they raise the risk of dehydration and decreased blood volume. Ultimately the result can be confusion, memory loss and even coma. Fasting is particularly dangerous for people with health conditions such as diabetes, low blood pressure or stomach ulcers" (Albertson 1996). Dehydration can occur in as little as one day.

If weight loss occurs, it may not only be from fat loss but also muscle. When muscle atrophies, the metabolism decreases, making weight gain inevitable after the end of the fast or any other diet. Also, the metabolism changes to reserve energy in case of another fast.

Fasting is neither safe nor effective nor cleansing, so do not do it. If your religion requires it at some point, find a way to alter your beliefs, even slightly, in the name of health.

L-Carnitine

L-Carnitine, an amino acid, has been sold on the premise that it enhances fat burning during exercise and improves athletic performance.

"Vukovich and others at Ball State University observed no changes in fat utilization during and after 60 minutes of cycle ergometer exercise at 70 percent of VO_2 $_{max}$ in response to L-carnitine supplementation. They concluded that there is an adequate amount of L-carnitine present within the mitochondria to support fat oxidation" (La Forge 1994). VO_2 $_{max}$ means aerobic capacity, the most amount of Calories your body can burn at one time (measured in ml O_2/kg body weight/minute). Mitochondria are known as the energy storehouses of the cell, or the place where food, including fat, is converted to energy.

University of Toledo researchers found "no significant improvement in 5K running performance in trained male runners after carnitine supplementation" (La Forge 1994).

Carnitine does aid in fat metabolism, but that does not mean that taking supplements—carnitine in excess—will help us to lose weight. In fact, it can be dangerous. There have been reports of supplementation causing serious blood sugar drops, leading to a hypoglycemic seizure and masking of heart disease symptoms.

A healthy diet supplies enough of the nutrient.

A lot of nutrients aid in fat metabolism, provide energy, and help to build muscle, but taking supplements will not make the process faster or greater. The body will only use what it needs, and the rest . . . becomes expensive urine.

Ginseng

Ginseng, an herb, has been tested in two different studies at Wayne State University to see if it matches up to its claims. Smith and colleagues tested a ginseng extract and found that in college-age women there were no significant effects on the women's metabolism or perceived effort (La Forge 1995).

Its claims include increasing energy and mental alertness. Although these have not been proven, hypertension, nervousness, and insomnia have been effects of ginseng consumption ($\geq$ 3 grams).

Here is another magical herb you can pass up.

Bee Pollen

A mixture of vitamins and organic compounds make up bee pollen. If it is good for flowers, it must be good for us. What?!

Along with vitamins and minerals per se, no credible studies have proven that bee pollen offers any ergogenic (work-enhancing) effect or induces a faster recovery from exercise (as claimed).

Regardless of bee pollen's effects, many people cannot take it due to allergy.

High-Protein/Amino Acid Consumption

Amino acids make up protein, which constitutes muscles and hormones among other functions. Both amino acid supplementation and excessive protein consumption are practiced as a form of dieting, exercise performance enhancement, and muscle building.

There exists a lot of research on whether or not athletes have a higher protein requirement than non-athletes. At least three studies, cited here, suggest that athletes do need more protein than the RDA (Celejowa and Homa 1970, Friedman and Lemon 1985, Yoshimura, et al. 1980). So does that mean athletes need to go out and spend a lot of money on amino acid supplements? No. As a matter of fact, most protein powders contain more milligrams of amino acids in one serving than we need in one day.

First, high-protein diets have negative side effects, such as negative water balance, excessive Calories, and decreased calcium storage. "Metabolism of protein requires more water than carbohydrate or fat and, therefore, as dietary protein increases increased water intake is recommended to minimize dehydration effects" (Lemon 1987). Since excessive intake of any type of Calories will be converted to fat, too much protein is again a concern. Too much fat storage can lead to obesity, which is associated with heart disease and diabetes. Increasing protein intake in excess of what is recommended has been proven to elevate calcium excretion (Allen, et al. 1972). If prolonged without calcium supplementation, osteoporosis could result.

The second reason you do not need to buy amino acid supplements is because adequate protein intake can be obtained by comprising 12-15% of the total daily Caloric consumption. When energy expenditure increases and protein needs increase, energy intake increases. If energy intake increases, and 12-15% of the Calories still come from protein, then the total protein intake will elevate, too. Besides, the average American diet, without supplements, includes 50% more protein than necessary anyway.

As for increasing muscle mass, the efficacy of protein in and of itself cannot enhance the process beyond what normally occurs. Similarly, aspartate, chromium, carnitine, boron, wheat germ oil, gamma hydroxy butyrate (GHB) and gamma oryzanol have no ergogenic effects (Stone 1994). The RDA for protein is .8 grams/kg/day. For athletes, it is approximately 1.2-1.5 kg/day.

To figure out your requirement, assuming you are either sedentary or a moderate exerciser, divide your weight (in pounds) by 2.2 then multiply that figure by .8. For example, a person weighing 220 pounds:

$$220/2.2 = 100 \text{ kg (kilograms)}$$

$$100 \text{ x } .8 = 80 \text{ grams}$$

This person needs 80 grams of protein per day.

Why take amino acids, anyway, if you have a small intestine? It does a fine job of breaking down proteins into amino acids.

High-protein diets have surged, again, after being popular in the '60s and '70s. Businesses claim that high-carbohydrate diets are harmful, which has never been proven. Regardless, people are losing weight on these diets and feeling good and it is no wonder. These diets control portions and Calories and emphasize eating vegetables and fruits throughout the day. That is what we nutritional counselors have been touting for years. Although the weight loss encourages people, high-protein diets can be harmful, as discussed earlier.

"Perhaps the most widely publicized problem incurred with amino acid supplements was the outbreak of the rare blood disorder eosinophilia-myalgia syndrome (EMS) in 1989. EMS is associated with a bad batch of the amino acid L-tryptophan, prescribed to eliminate insomnia. An estimated 1,500 Americans are known to have come down with the disease (Green 1992).

Tyrosine, another amino acid, has led to side effects such as a rapid decrease in blood pressure.

There is no valid research which suggests that a high protein diet and/or any type of amino acid supplementation aids in exercise performance, weight loss, or muscle gain.

Sports Drinks

Gatorade, probably the most widely drunk sports drink, provides energy, electrolytes (e.g., sodium, potassium), and water during exercise sessions. Other sports drinks provide similar benefits, Exceed probably being the best.

In this section, rather than compare and contrast sports drinks, I would like to help you decide whether or not you need them.

If your exercise session lasts less than two hours, you will only need a lot of water. Above that time period, you will need some Calories for energy, assuming that you are exercising *continuously* for more than two hours (e.g., biking counts, playing in a baseball game does not count). Fruit juice, simply, can provide the carbohydrates that sports drinks do. Choose one without sugar added, and then mix one part of it with five parts water to dilute it. For example: every cup of juice should be mixed with five cups of water. If you need something to fill you up during longer exercise sessions, a banana or trail mix, for example, can be carted easily. For ultra-long events, something with fat in it will be needed to prevent "hitting the wall." In that case, nuts or trail mix can be useful.

As for electrolytes, a healthy meal before the session will provide enough. Even endurance athletes do not need to consume electrolytes during exercise, because their bodies are trained enough not to allow too much to be released with water in sweat. As a result, the actual blood concentration of sodium, chloride, and potassium rises, negating the need for replacement during exercise and making water even more important than sports drinks or juice. Although, ultra-long events require these minerals during participation, which can be acquired via juice and food.

A healthy meal after an exercise session can replace lost electrolytes, enhance recovery, and replace glycogen (stored glucose).

Sports Bars

I feel the same way about sports bars as I do sports drinks. They are an expensive means of obtaining nutrients that you might not even need.

If your exercise session will last less than two hours, you will neither need a sports bar before nor during exercise. A healthy meal a couple of hours before your workout can provide enough nutrients to keep you going. Still, you will need to drink a lot of water during exercise.

As for long or ultra-long events, juice and food can provide energy and electrolytes as needed.

After exercise, a healthy meal provides a much better means, than sports bars, for replenishing the body.

Creatine

Creatine, synthesized in the body from amino acids, is part of creatine phosphate, which has importance in muscle contraction. Manufacturers of this product claim it increases creatine phosphate in muscles, improves energy, and stimulates muscle growth.

Some research suggests that creatine supplements increase power in short-term, high-intensity exercise and increases weight (from water or protein).

Although this nutrient has substantial claims, let the scientists study it for a few more years before you run to your local health food store. The sprinters often lose the races to the store, while lingerers often win, because the latter waits until further research demonstrates that previous research is in fact true and a product is in fact safe. As for creatine supplementation, long-term effects are still unknown.

Caffeine

We all know what caffeine is, right? It is a drug, a stimulant found in some of our foods, such as coffee, colas, chocolate, and some diet pills. So, how did it make its way into my book? Well, since it is an "upper," athletes use it for supposed ergogenic and fat-burning benefits. Those claims have not been substantiated in clinical trials, where subjects consumed caffeine before exercise.

"Graf (1950) has reported on experiments in Germany during World War II to find stimulants suitable for improving physical and mental efficiency in combating the stressful conditions of war. It was found that, although caffeine was a strong mental stimulant, it resulted in a very undesirable impairment of motor coordination (in target shooting, writing, and simulated auto driving). There was also a hangover effect, in which mental efficiency, after having been improved, fell off below normal values from one to three hours after the stimulant was taken" (deVries and Housh 1994).

More recently, caffeine was tested to see whether or not it would create an emphasis toward fat utilization during endurance exercise, thus sparing glucose (sugar).

Wilcox (1990) summarized that "the majority of the studies evaluating substrate utilization during a fixed interval (ranging from 60 to 120 minutes) of running or cycling find no evidence of enhanced fat utilization following caffeine consumption." Therefore, it still has not been proven that caffeine enhances fat utilization during exercise.

Even if caffeine does enhance exercise performance, it might also cause cramping, dehydration, nervousness, nausea, headaches, and muscle tremors—all side effects. How can you perform well with those symptoms?

Just drink a lot of water.

Hydro-K Energy*

Hydro-K Energy offers a water pill that contains herbs and potassium. "Take with water," the manufacturers emphasize. A water pill is not a pill that contains water. It is a pill that is used to make you lose water—it is a diuretic. When you lose water, you lose weight. But you also lose potassium, which is why potassium was added to this pill.

There are different types of diuretics. The most powerful ones inhibit salt and water reabsorption in the kidneys by as much as 25%. Therefore, diuretics intensify urine production and excretion. Coffee, tea, alcohol, excitement, and worry are more or less mild diuretics. More powerful diuretic drugs are often prescribed in heart disease and kidney disease to prevent or overcome the accumulation of excess fluids in the body tissues. Some of these diuretics contain mercury, which has a specific effect on kidney cells.

Since the taking of a diuretic increases water excretion, it causes sudden weight loss. A person who fails to distinguish between loss of body fat and loss of water may see this as a desirable effect and start using diuretics for this purpose. But because the only loss induced is water loss, the only achievement gained is temporary dehydration and possibly excessive potassium loss.

Overfat people are more likely to use diuretics for weight loss and more likely to become dehydrated due to their *smaller* percentage of body water than people of normal weight. The effects of dehydration include the inability of the body to regulate its temperature, and muscle cramps, nausea, and decreased blood volume (which hinders physical performance).

The effects of potassium deficiency warrant the replacement of the mineral while taking diuretics, unless it is a potassium-sparing diuretic. Some of the effects of potassium deficiency include nervous disorders, insomnia, constipation, slow and irregular heartbeat, and muscle damage. When a deficiency of potassium impairs glucose metabolism, energy is no longer available to the muscles, which become more or less paralyzed. Also, the sodium content of the heart and muscles increases.

Early symptoms of potassium deficiency include general weakness and impairment of neuromuscular function, poor reflexes, and soft, sagging muscles. In adolescents, acne can result; in older persons, dry skin may occur.

Another water pill manufacturer also sells a "meal replacement shake." Nothing can replace a meal, except a meal. Meals should not be skipped or exchanged with a low-Calorie filler. Your body needs food, so eat— nutritiously!

Bicker Lads*

Bicker Lads sells energy supplements, which I found in a nutrition store.

Turn "fat to energy." Remember that exercise can turn fat to energy and it is free.

One-Day Diet*

"Lose weight around the clock." This company also sells supplements, which I found in a nutrition store. The diet contains chromium, amino acids, minerals, fiber, water pills (herbs), and a high percentage (more than 100%) of the RDA for vitamins.

If you exercise (including strength training) every day, you will keep your metabolism at a higher level than if you do not exercise, and you will burn Calories around the clock and lose weight. Also, exercise will benefit you in many other ways than a diet will. The name of this product, in and of itself, should turn you off. Diets do not work.

Whey

Whey is the watery portion of milk—what is left after casein (milk protein) is removed. Manufacturers sell whey as a special kind of protein for bodybuilders, among others. Although whey has *some* protein, why not have all of the milk or any other dairy product, which provide a lot more protein and other nutrients than just whey?

Whey occurs naturally and should cause no harm when consumed, unless you are allergic to it. Just contemplate whether or not you really need this type of supplement.

Phosphate Loading

In the past, sodium phosphate has been administered orally as an ergogenic aid. "The procedure normally involves ingesting approximately 600 to 1,000 milligrams of sodium phosphate, four to six times per day for three to six days prior to exercise" (deVries and Housh 1994).

Its effects on endurance performance and strength tests have shown favorable results in some experiments and not in others. Since the research is still inconclusive, more tests need to be performed to prove phosphate loading is actually beneficial.

Amphetamines (Benzedrine)

"An amphetamine, in all its various form (primarily d-amphetamine sulfate and its European relative Pervitin), is a sympathomimetic amine [a type of ammonia which mimics nervous system action], and it is used by the medical profession as a central nervous system stimulant. Pharmacology texts warn against its use as a remedy for sleepiness or fatigue or to increase capacity for work because: 1) there is a danger of addiction, 2) it removes the warning of impending overstrain, 3) its vasopressor effects are undesirable, and 4) cases of collapse have been reported. Obviously, this discussion is academic, as the use of such drugs by athletes is to be strongly discouraged" (deVries and Housh 1994).

The effects of amphetamines on fatigue, coordination, strength, and endurance have been tested, but also show inconclusive results in various studies. Even if the drug proved helpful for a particular athlete, the risks involved stand much higher than the benefits.

Wheat-Germ Oil

The vitamin E, fatty acids, and alcohol in wheat-germ oil provide the health benefits that many researchers and manufacturers claim. Unfortunately, many of the valid studies have not shown significant ergogenic effects.

Sharman, et al. (1973) performed a well-controlled study on adolescent human swimmers, which showed no effects due to vitamin E supplementation.

Slim Tea*

Slim Tea claims that it is "for a healthier and prettier you." It contains Tze-Bei tea and malve verticellata—an herb—that supposedly curbs one's appetite and therefore aids in weight loss. Folks, tea will not make you prettier. No kidding? Then, how do they get away with making this claim? Remember that the FDA still has not tested all herbs. It is possible that this tea includes one that the FDA has not tested, yet.

Why not lose weight by eating properly and exercising? To a certain extent, exercise curbs your appetite while you burn Calories. What a bonus! As for eating, you should learn portion *control*, rather than using a drug or herb to control your psychological reasons for overeating.

Since I first wrote this book, the ob1—obesity gene— was discovered. Obese people can now blame their excessive eating habits on genetics.

Get-Trim*

"It changed my life and if it can change mine, it can change yours," one woman raves. Get-Trim contains aloe vera, an appetite suppressant (supposedly). That is interesting: an appetite suppressant that gives you nice-looking skin.

Other testimonials included ones made by celebrities. Why should we believe *them*? We should not. Just because they have entertained us, does not mean that they have credibility in the fitness industry.

I have not read any credible studies on this plant relating to appetite suppression. Do not try this product.

Be Slimmer*

This multi-level marketing company sells products that contain aloe vera, in addition to colloidal ("purified") silver and other ingredients. They claim that their product helps to balance the body's chemistry, increase energy, cure *many* ailments, and boost the immune system. Also, they believe many Americans are mineral deficient, because the plants grown these days lack nutrients due to poor soil quality. If Americans are mineral deficient, it is because they do not consume the minimum requirement of five servings of produce per day and they consume empty-Calorie (no nutritional value) foods that require the body's stored or circulating nutrients to digest them.

Be Slimmer admits that they purposely omit nutrient values (e.g., milligrams of vitamin C per serving) from their packaging labels. They say that other companies who show the values pad them with added synthetic nutrients. In other words, Be Slimmer has something to hide.

Wait for *many* valid research studies on America's soil, colloidal silver, and aloe vera, before trying Be Slimmer. Be skeptical, especially when a product sounds like a cure-all.

Lecithin

The liver manufactures lecithin, an emulsifier (aids in fat digestion), which constitutes cell membranes. As you can guess, since lecithin aids in fat digestion, manufacturers add it to their high-fat foods to make consumers think the food will digest properly and the fat will not be absorbed. Also, lecithin pills exist.

You might also see choline and inositol, B vitamins, when reading about lecithin. Among other functions, they help to make up lecithin. Making an effort to consume these vitamins through supplements, for example, will not necessarily get your body to make more lecithin. When consuming a healthy diet, you are bound to get enough choline and inositol, since they are found in many foods.

Since lecithin is a non-essential nutrient (do not need in diet), we do not need to look for foods that contain it. As a matter of fact, it can be toxic in large doses, causing sweating, loss of appetite, and gastrointestinal upset.

As for now, do not worry if you see lecithin in a list of ingredients. Just do not buy it in pill form or think that it makes a product healthier.

Spur-U-Leaner*

Spur-U-Leaner, containing microalgae, is sold at juice stores as an additive. One store claims that it provides energy, because it offers B vitamins. Real food, like whole grain bread, meats, eggs, and legumes also have B vitamins. You do not need to become a sea erchant to get your daily requirement of B vitamins and therefore to have energy.

Ego Boost*

Ego Boost is an "energy drink" that won't actually give you more energy, but it will make you think more highly of yourself. In fact, you won't have to drink it; just buying it means that you already have a big ego. Maybe you don't even have to buy it; just thinking about wanting an ego boost means that you already have an ego.

A client and I made this up.

Viva Grim*

"... for fast pick-up—safe as coffee ... same amount of caffeine as two cups of coffee ... so you'll get the pick up you need to get to the gym and pump up." Why not just drink coffee, then? It probably costs less.

Anyway, remember what I wrote earlier on caffeine. Do not use it as an ergogenic aid or a boost to get you to the gym. Instead, use a motivational tactic to get you to the gym, like intrinsic and extrinsic rewards. Intrinsic, something intangible, includes feeling well mentally and physically, for example; and extrinsic, something tangible, includes taking yourself to the movies or buying a new outfit. Do not ever reward yourself with food. Only think of food as nourishment—not a reward, not a crutch, not a punishment.

Other non-effective supplements

Other non-effective supplements, meaning valid research has not supported their claims, include antioxidants (vitamins C, E, and beta carotene), magnesium, medium-chain triglycerides, and omega-3 fatty acids. Examples of the unsupported claims include increased muscle growth, increased fat burning, ergogenic effects, and decreased muscle damage from unwanted oxidation.

Although quackery exists with these nutrients, they are still an important part of a healthy diet.

Nutritional products are the ones with which I want you to be most careful (after drugs/medicine). They can hurt you a lot more than an exercise product, since they affect you systemically. Be very careful! Research it as much as you would your child's future school, your future employer, a school paper, or a used car. Get the picture? Do not just throw anything down your throat. Your digestive tract is a portal to health, not a garbage disposal.

References

Albertson E. 1996. "Fasting." *Am Health* July/August; 65.

Allen LH, Oddoye EA, Margen S. 1979. "Protein-Induced Hypercalciuria: a Longer Term Study." *Am J Clin Nut* 32; 741-49.

Celejowa I, Homa M. 1970. "Food Intake, Nitrogen and Energy Balance in Polish Weight Lifters during a Training Camp." *Nut Metab* 12; 259-74.

deVries HA, and TJ Housh. 1994. *Physiology of Exercise*. Madison: Brown & Benchmark.

Dunne LJ. 1990. *Nutrition Almanac*. New York: McGraw-Hill NY.

Friedman JE, Lemon PWR. 1985. "Effect of Protein Intake and Endurance Exercise on Daily Protein Requirements (Abstract)." *Med Sci Sports Ex* 17; 231-32.

Graf O. 1950. "Increase of Efficiency by Means of Pharmaceutics (Stimulants)." *Germ Aviat Med, WW II* 2; 1080.

Green R. 1992. "Amino Acids: Heading for Drug Status?" *Am Fit* November/December; 60-61.

Hallmark M, et al. 1996. "Effects of Chromium and Resistive Training on Muscle Strength and Body Composition." *Med Sci Sports Ex* 28; 139-44.

La Forge R. 1995. "Research Reports." *IDEA* October; 53.

La Forge R. 1994. "Exercise and L-Carnitine Supplementation." *IDEA* October; 52.

Lemon PWR. 1987. "Protein and Exercise: Update 1987." *Med Sci Sports Ex* 19; S179-S190.

Miller M. 1997. "Weight Loss Firm Settles Ad Suit." *San Diego Union Tribune* May 30; C-1,8.

Sharman IM, Down MG, Sen RN. 1973. "The Effects of Training and Vitamin E Supplementation on the Performance of Adolescent Swimmers." *Brit J Sports Med* 7; 27-30.

Stone MH. 1994. "Weight Gain and Weight Loss." *Essentials of Strength Training and Conditioning.* Champaign: Human Kinetics.

Wilcox AR. 1990. "Caffeine and Endurance Performance." *Gatorade Sports Sci Exch* 3; 26.

Yoshimura H, Inoue T, Yamada T, Shivaki K. 1980. "Anemia during Hard Physical Training (Sports Anemia) and its Causal Mechanism with Special Reference to Protein Nutrition." *World Rev Nut Diet* 35; 1-86.

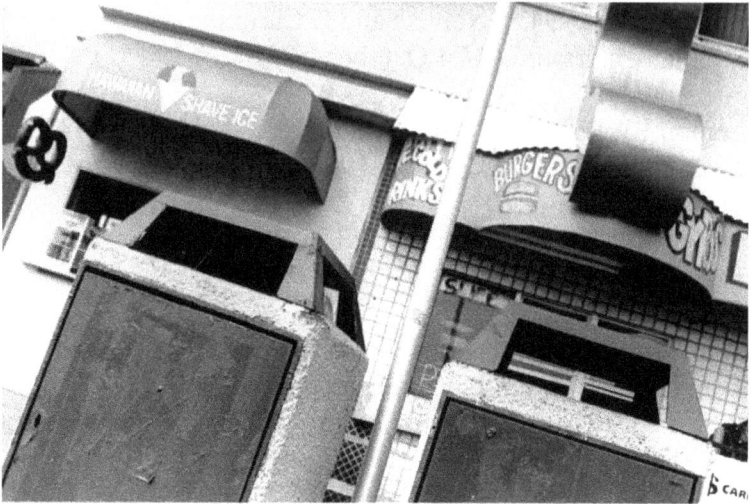

Dump bad habits.

San Diego, California

CHAPTER 3

THE MEDIA:
BOOKS, VIDEOTAPES, MAGAZINES,
AND TV SHOWS

This chapter highlights media sources used to feed you fitness information. Unfortunately, there is a lot of misinformation out there. People write books to lure you to their "perfect workout" and video exercise demonstrations, and publish magazines that contain advertisements for many of America's useless fitness products and services.

Below are the media sources I researched. Some of the books may have been updated since I first researched them, but if they contained contraindicated exercises at the time that the books were contemporary, then they probably are still not accurate resources, unless a qualified expert were hired as a consultant.

BOOKS

Perfect Parts

This book is one of several written by Joyce Vedral, PhD, and I might say she looks great at 50+ years old. She really does look fantastic for her age, but that does not necessarily mean that she knows a lot about the body and gives credible exercise and nutrition advice, right?

When I first leafed through this book, I noticed a lot of exercises demonstrated (by her) that were either contraindicated or not quite done with proper form. Also, I wondered why her posture in many of the photographs appeared more like poses—bodybuilding and modeling. The public needs to know how to perform an exercise properly without necessarily getting turned on.

After finishing my critique of the book, I questioned, "In what does she have her PhD, anyway?" Certainly, it's not in exercise physiology. Her educational experience was not listed in the book.

A few weeks later, I was at the bookstore, again, but this time scanning the self-help/psychology books. Guess who writes those types of books, too. Same woman. As it turns out, her doctorate is in English! In the psychology books her educational experience was listed.

If you pick up an exercise or nutrition book and see that the author has a PhD, look to see in what the degree is. If it does not say, then it probably is not in an exercise-related field. Choose a book that is written by someone who has a health-related degree (whether BS, MS, PhD, RD, MPH), not simply a PhD in anything.

Body Engineering

Body Engineering, copyrighted in 1997, had many contraindicated exercises and ones that were simply done wrong. I was surprised, since the book was written at the time of my research.

When choosing a fitness book, check to see what year it was written. Exercise physiologists have learned a lot in the last ten and especially twenty years. Hopefully, recently-written books will have updated information.

Getting Stronger

Getting Stronger, copyrighted in 1986, also has many contraindicated exercises and ones that were done wrong. I was not surprised, though, after looking at what year it was written.

Stretching

Stretching was copyrighted in 1980 and written by Bob Anderson. In it there are many contraindicated stretches and ones that are done wrong. As a matter of fact, this book is referenced *a lot* in other publications, including stretching charts that are placed on a wall for reference. That worries me. Too many people are seeing and using these outdated stretches.

Even if you have a reference of safe and effective stretches and exercises, how do you know which are right for you?

Ugh! This is my least favorite book, because I see it everywhere and I wonder what fueled its longevity. I cannot believe that it is still available. In my opinion, this book is the cockroach of fitness books—it has no purpose, exists everywhere, appears in places I would never expect, and is a pain in the ass to get rid of.

The Gold's Gym Training Encyclopedia

The Gold's Gym Training Encyclopedia, copyrighted in 1984, contains many contraindicated exercises and ones that are done wrong. As a reminder, contraindicated means that an exercise is risky and can cause injury. What I mean by "ones that are done wrong" is that some of the demonstrated exercises are good, but are not quite done properly. For example, the model has his wrists extended when they should be straight.

It is really important for exercises to be demonstrated properly, because a learner who duplicates the movement should be doing it correctly. Many exercise programs have been stopped due to injuries caused by poor form. This tends to make people think that exercising is not worth the risk of injury. Then, they become part of the too many of those who will not exercise and therefore are obese and sick with lifestyle-related diseases. Doing exercises properly eliminates the risk of injury.

During the twelve years that I offered personal fitness training, I had a rule: no one gets hurt on my watch. And, no one did.

Joe Weider's Ultimate Bodybuilding

Joe Weider's Ultimate Bodybuilding was copyrighted in 1989 and contains many contraindicated exercises and ones that are done wrong.

Arnold Schwarzenegger Encyclopedia of Modern Bodybuilding

Arnold Schwarzenegger Encyclopedia of Modern Bodybuilding was copyrighted in 1985. I guess it is not so modern anymore, is it? It contains many contraindicated exercises and ones that are done wrong.

Enter the Zone

Enter the Zone, written by Barry Sears, PhD, promotes a high-protein diet. As I discussed earlier in the book, a high-protein diet is not only unhealthy but also not what Americans need to lose weight. Americans are overweight, because they still consume too many Calories and do not exercise enough.

For many years, nutrition counselors (including myself) have recommended a diet that obtains 55-58% of daily Calories from carbohydrates, 12-15% from protein, and less than or equal to 30% from fat. Since many Americans are still overweight, "experts" search for other, perhaps more effective, Caloric ratios. It is not that the above ratio is ineffective; it is that many people are still not following it, consuming too many Calories, and exercising too little.

As for exercise, Dr. Sears thinks that the main goal is to burn fat. "If you only want to burn excess body fat for energy—that is, if you're less concerned with building strength or lean body mass—then aerobic exercise is for you." One type of exercise offers no greater benefit over the other. Everyone needs both aerobic and anaerobic (strength) training. As for weight loss, aerobic may burn fat immediately, but since strength training can increase muscle size, it can result in more fat being burned at rest than without such training.

69

Barry Sears has his PhD in biochemistry. That is impressive, but it is not exercise physiology.

VIDEOTAPES

Jane Fonda's Workout Videos

Jane Fonda's name has coincided with aerobics for many years. She started with high-impact aerobics tapes, which are too hard on the body, and more recently made a *Personal Trainer Series*. As a matter of fact, the high-impact, very outdated aerobics tapes are still on the rental shelves (at the time of original research). Who is borrowing them? Should those tapes be "recalled?" They can not only hurt untrained people but also experienced exercisers who watch the tapes at home on their hard floors (carpeted or not). Even on the most technologically advanced, cushioned aerobics floor, high-impact aerobics creates a lot of skeletal pounding.

I would rather see a *Personal Trainer Series* produced and demonstrated by a qualified personal trainer. This series includes "Jane's personal health and exercise guidelines for eating right and staying lean and healthy for life." Eating right? Hmm. That is interesting, coming from someone with a (past?) eating disorder. ". . . her own fitness training techniques." In my opinion, you should not use her guidelines or techniques. Follow American College of Sports Medicine's (ACSM) guidelines on exercise prescription and testing, Food and Drug Administration (FDA), and American Dietetic Association. They are the ones who write guidelines based on peer-reviewed research. You cannot follow one person's guidelines, just because it worked for her.

Jane Fonda's Workout—*Sport Aid*—touts: "This video . . . contains exercise intended to reduce the risk of

70

sports injuries." The best way to avoid injuries is by avoiding her tapes. In one, it shows her doing aerobics with wrist weights on. As I wrote earlier in the book, using weights during aerobic exercise can alter your gait and negatively stress the joints. On the cover of two of the videos she has one knee hyperflexed (too bent), which overstretches the knee ligaments, leaving them weak and prone to injury.

Others

Generally, avoid tapes that star an actress/actor, model, or sports figure. Choose ones made by people, such as Kathy Smith and Denise Austin, who are actually exercise experts; they obtain exercise-related degrees. Also, the Reebok videos are very good.

The Abs of Steel and related videos, by Tamilee Webb, may demonstrate proper exercises, but spend too much time on a particular area. With the exception of certain athletes, no one needs to do abdominal exercises for 20 minutes each session. The minimum amount of time one needs to spend strength training the whole body is 20 minutes, twice a week. I tell my clients to spend more time exercising aerobically, to lose excess fat, than trying to spot reduce. Besides, you will never see a toned muscle if you still have fat covering it.

The following is a list of stars with their own videotapes that you should avoid: Daisy Fuentes—spokesperson/MTV personality, Elle Macpherson-model, Cindy Crawford-model, and Cher-actress/singer.

Richard Simmons, who is great at catering to the severely overweight and unconditioned, offers safe routines.

EXERCISE TV SHOWS

Body Shaping

Body Shaping can be seen on ESPN and includes aerobics and strength training. When I was watching, there were a few contraindicated abdominal exercises demonstrated. Usually the area of the body that contraindicated abdominal exercises hurt is the lower back. Abdominal exercises are recommended not only to strengthen the abdominal muscles but also to help support the lower back. When contraindicated exercises are performed, the back is weakened rather than strengthened.

One might find, while watching (notice I do not say following along with) these shows that the women have very large chests. Artificially large? I do not know. Yes, I do have a small chest. No, I do not have "large-chest envy." I simply do not like to see exercise used as an avenue to get people to tune into a channel, open a book, or read a magazine to see "pretty" girls (or men). The more natural (i.e., without plastic surgery) professionals look, the more likely they practice a healthy lifestyle and exercise in a safe and effective manner. Therefore, they are appropriate people to follow.

Also, the buff women and men whom I see on these TV shows probably do not attract the population who needs exercise the most. I have spoken with a lot of overweight people who have told me that instructors who look like bodybuilders intimidate them, let alone the fact that the overweight people are unwilling to exercise in the same gym as bodybuilders. Many overweight people think that they could never look like the instructors, so why bother trying what they are teaching?

The strength training exercises that are taught on these shows require equipment that most people do not have, such as free weights and squat rack. Do you think

72

people will go out and buy them and set them up in front of their television? No.

Lastly, TV instructors cannot assume that their whole audience can do every exercise. Similarly, people cannot assume that an exercise is safe for them. Each person requires their own, unique program and therefore should not follow a routine of generic exercises. Consulting a qualified personal trainer is the best way to know what you need. Are these TV instructors qualified?

Kiana's Flex Appeal

On this show, I saw some contraindicated exercises demonstrated and ones that were done wrong.

The guy on the show said, "Sometimes I let my ego get in the way and don't do the exercises right" (because of trying to lift too heavy). He does not do them right even when his ego isn't in the way. Don't follow someone who chooses ego over health.

Cory Everson's Total Body Workout

On this show, I saw exercises that could injure the back, wrists, and knees.

MAGAZINES

Unfortunately, there are no health magazines that I like. *Health*, formerly *American Health*, used to be fantastic, but it went downhill, especially after becoming a women's magazine. I am not impressed with *Shape*, *Weight Watchers*, and *Self*, either.

Also, I am not impressed with what is probably the most popular bodybuilding magazine: *Joe Weider's Muscle and Fitness Magazine*. First, it is loaded with advertisements for nutritional supplements—enough to fuel one chapter of this book. Second, it shows photos of people demonstrating exercises improperly, which could injure the wrists and knees, among other joints. Arnold Schwarzenegger was highlighted in the issue I read and was among those doing exercises wrong. Lastly, the magazine promotes competitive bodybuilding, which is unhealthy in and of itself. It appears that not only is being on steroids the norm in this magazine but also radically changing one's diet to lose as much body fat and water, as possible, to have the skin close to the muscle. A lot of competitors dehydrate themselves in order to enhance muscle definition.

To obtain the latest fitness facts and to consider ideas for *your* ideal workout and eating habits, learn how the body responds to exercise and proper nutrition. Ultimately, *you* (and a personal trainer and registered dietitian) will design your *own* program for wellness.

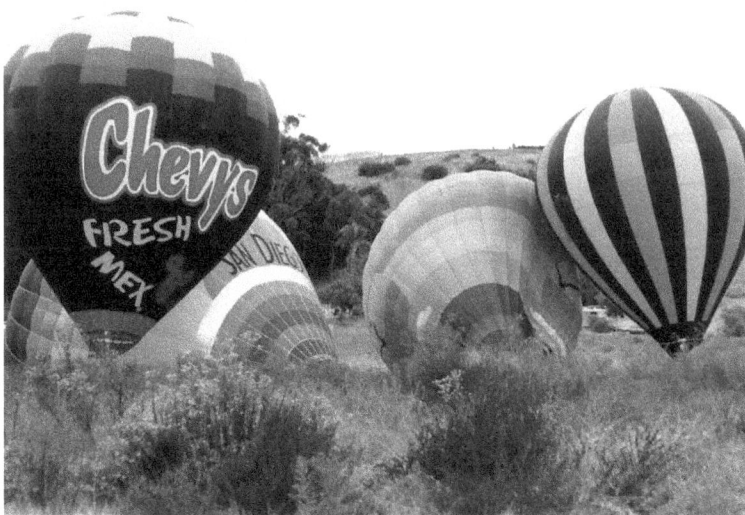

Balloons aren't the only things filled with a lot of hot air.

San Diego, California

CHAPTER 4

FITNESS "PROFESSIONALS"

America, especially California, is home to a lot of people claiming to be fitness professionals. So who is, actually? The following list includes people, types of people, and businesses with employees whose credibility should be questioned.

Mara Hoskin-Thomas

"Workout for women focuses on losing inches, not adding muscle." Why not add muscle? Oh. Getting bulky and looking like a man scares women. I have news for you: A very small percentage of women can get bulky naturally—without steroids—from exercising. What does it take to get bulky? Be a man; be Black, preferably, since their genetics make them more likely to get muscular than a Caucasian; perform more than three sets of each exercise, ten or fewer reps. max. (the most you can do at a given weight), more than one exercise per muscle group, three times a week; and be young.

Muscle has a high demand for energy, therefore the more muscle you have the more Calories you burn. We should concern ourselves more with *losing* muscle than gaining too much. We lose muscle as we age, but we can control the rate and amount by exercising, especially strength training. When muscle mass decreases, the body expends fewer Calories. If we continue to eat our usual amount and do not exercise, fat stores increase.

Mara's program highlights working the lower abs, attaining fast results, and strength training on six consecutive days to disallow muscle rest. You know how I feel about the first two points. As for the third, muscles require 48 hours to rest and repair, otherwise they cannot adapt to the stress they receive and become stronger, healthier, and bigger. Mara's objective: do not let the muscles get bigger. How counterintuitive. Women and men need muscle growth to decrease (indirectly) fat stores and to help ensure strength and an independent lifestyle as they age.

The article written about this lady's "cutting-edge" techniques listed her credentials, which do not include a bachelor's degree in an exercise-related field.

24 Hour Nautilus Fitness Centers

The Nautilus I visited was in Sunnyvale, California. They told me that five out of the eighteen trainers had exercise-related degrees. Be sure that you would hire one of those five.

I asked for help from one of those without a degree. I purposely did some things wrong to see if he would catch them. In one exercise, I had my wrists extended, and in another I had my head tilted forward. He did not catch either one. It is really important that an exerciser has everything just right to avoid injury. I asked this guy about free weights and he said, "Using machines can make you stronger than free weights." That is not true. At any given intensity, machines and free weights will have the same strength result. Lastly, he touched me without asking for my permission. That may seem like no big deal, but it would make many people uncomfortable, especially those who have suffered physical abuse.

Finally, this fitness center did not have any trainers on the floor to answer questions. At least one trainer should always be circulating to correct exercisers who may be putting themselves at risk. You would want assistance if you were doing something wrong, right?

Fitness USA

The Fitness USA gym I went to was in Sunnyvale, California. It had eight personal trainers. No one would tell me how many held a degree. As a matter of fact, one exclaimed, "Trainers don't need a degree to teach you how to use the equipment!" Oh, my gosh. Excuse me! That's not all that trainers do.

The trainer who helped me did not have a degree and it was obvious. She was so bad that I was embarrassed for her. Also, she is one of the many who give trainers a reputation for not actually knowing a lot about exercise. First, she had me fill out a medical questionnaire and write any diseases I have. I told her that I have celiac disease, a gluten intolerance, which I do. She just said, "Oh." I could tell that she had no idea what gluten was, which is alright, but she should have asked me. It is really important for a trainer to ask a lot of questions about a disease, because the disease may dictate which exercises should be performed or avoided. Second, she tried taking my measurements in the middle of the weight room. Although I am not that modest, I declined. I wanted to prove my point that it was unprofessional. Third, she did not teach me how to use the equipment or how to do the exercises. She just suggested, "Do 12 repetitions," then walked away. She never watched any of my sets and therefore could not correct my form, even though I did it right. I wasn't going to risk hurting myself "off camera."

The last problem I had with the gym was the aerobics instructor. I noticed that during his class, he was doing high-impact aerobics, while the rest were doing very low impact. He was not paying attention to his students.

I considered going to every local gym that is part of a national chain to critique their trainers, but I stopped at two. I decided that two gyms were enough for me to make my point: hire trainers with an exercise-related (college) degree. Being certified by the gym or a fitness organization is not good enough. There is too much that one needs to know about the body to forgo a college education.

One of the reasons why my colleagues and I are so knowledgeable is that we conducted an enormous amount of exercise testing, including stress tests. A stress test is a diagnostic exam to determine how the heart responds to exercise; the patient is usually on a treadmill. Conducting exercise tests is an important tool in understanding exercise, how to teach it, and how to design exercise conditioning programs. This is why:

$$x \text{ certifications} \neq \text{a degree}$$

TV Guide

Issue June 14-20, 1997, was a "Special Fitness Issue." It included "exercise secrets and diet tips from TV's buffest bods." Remember that a buff body does not mean a knowledgeable brain or a healthy body. Follow tips from qualified fitness professionals, not celebrities.

About four personal trainers to the stars were highlighted, too. I liked what they had to say, but there was a photo of one in a lunge position with his front knee forward of his ankle, which puts a lot of negative stress on the knee. I was surprised that he did not know how to lunge properly and I worried that he was not teaching his clients correctly.

A celebrity trainer does not necessarily make one a qualified trainer. Credentials. Credentials. Credentials. Always look for credentials.

Chiropractors

Chiropractors, although not *medical* doctors, obtain a doctorate of chiropractic (DC). Chiropractic is a "science which utilizes the recuperative powers of the body and the relationship between the musculoskeletal structures and functions of the body, particularly of the spinal column and the nervous system, in the restoration and maintenance of health" (Stedman 1982). I am sure the chiropractic field has its own definition, different from a medical dictionary, from which each chiropractor makes one's own interpretation.

These individual interpretations are, in part, what bring so much controversy to the chiropractic field. Many chiropractors believe that if any of the vertebrae (back bones) is out of line, it interferes with the brain's ability to communicate with the rest of the body by way of the spinal nerves. They believe this, in turn, can cause diseases.

Critics in the National Association for Chiropractic Medicine (NACM), including chiropractor Daniel Futch and the medical community, say "the wide appeal of adjustments to treat organic illness lies in the placebo effect of hands-on treatment and the easy-to-understand concept of the spine as a source of all ills. They also point to aggressive marketing as a sign that the field is not responsible" (Bredin 1993). Other critics agree that chiropractic sells itself as a means for curing a wide variety of illnesses—cures which scientific medicine has not proven.

Other concerns the NACM have include neck adjustments. Although the National Chiropractic Mutual Insurance Company (NCMIC) says the risky procedure results in complications between "[one in] 1 million and one in 10 million" (Bredin 1993), NACM is still concerned. They believe chiropractors should concentrate on the *lower* back for adjustments.

The following includes situations in which a chiropractor *cannot* help (Bredin 1993):

1. You have a systemic ailment that affects the entire body, such as arthritis.
2. You have a bone disease or bone infection.
3. You have a history of steroid use (steroids can make the bones weak and prone to fractures).
4. You have symptoms of cardiovascular disease.
5. You are taking anticoagulant drugs (they interfere with blood clotting and make chiropractic a risky business).

Chiropractors and other doctors use x-rays, often, to diagnose back pain. Unfortunately, x-rays cannot diagnose all back ailments, especially if disks, muscles, and ligaments cause them. The following includes situations in which you *would* need an x-ray (Klein and Sobel 1993):

1. You are over 50, since people in this age group are more likely to have osteoporosis, compression fractures of the spine, or malignancies.
2. You have had a recent fall or car accident, either of which could cause a fracture.
3. You have numbness or weakness of the kind associated with herniated disks, because these symptoms can also be caused by malignancies.
4. You have ever had cancer.
5. You have unexplained weight loss, which might be the result of cancer.
6. You have abused drugs or alcohol, and may be unaware of injuries sustained while intoxicated.
7. You have used corticosteroids, which may cause osteoporosis or susceptibility to infection.
8. You have a fever, which might indicate a spinal abscess.
9. Your pain lasts for more than a month, even in the absence of any of the symptoms above.

Even through all of the controversy, there seems to be universal agreement that chiropractors are most helpful in relieving minor or moderate low-back or neck pain, when they use gentle forms of manipulation and recommend exercise and stress management.

I listed chiropractors in this chapter, because they treat, diagnose, and suggest exercises for back problems. And, of course, they are controversial.

After many years of skepticism and back pain, I challenged a chiropractor to change my opinion and eliminate my back pain. He definitely succeeded on both accounts, because he was a credible, professional chiropractor who suggested a realistic treatment plan.

What credentials give a fitness professional credibility? Fitness professionals, especially personal fitness trainers, should have at least a bachelor's degree in an exercise-related field that includes nutrition education.

References

Bredin A. 1993. "The Chiropractic Controversy." *Men's Fitness* May; 110-113.

Klein AC, Sobel D. 1993. "Put an End to Back Pain." *AmHealth* September; 48-52.

Stedman T. 1982. *Stedman's Medical Dictionary*. London: Williams & Wilkins.

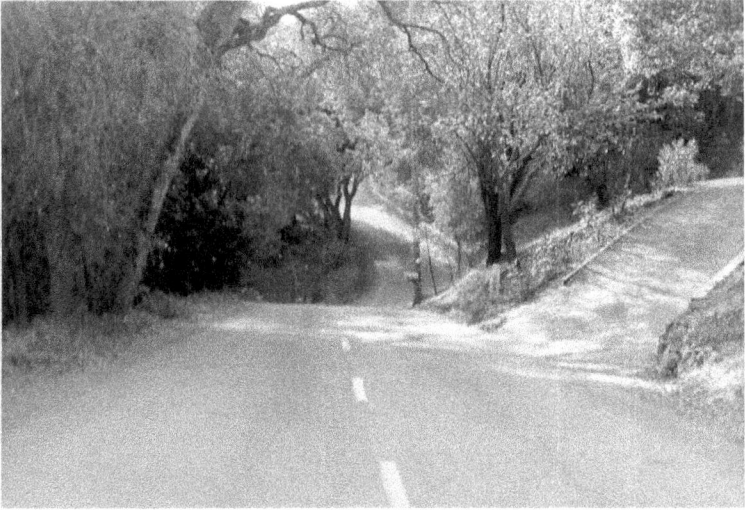

Choose the healthy path.

Cupertino, California

CHAPTER 5

MEDICAL TREATMENTS:

SURGERY/DRUGS

Beware of medically-supervised weight loss programs. It might sound good to have a doctor watch over you and offer advice, but usually these types of programs require you to take medication. So what? To lose weight, you need to burn more Calories than you are consuming, which requires eating in moderation and exercising, not finding some magical pill that suppresses your appetite or burns cellulite. Healthy lifestyle habits, not drugs, should be what you pursue. I will say that there exists an exception, i.e. a small population of people who might need weight-loss medication, but I will not suggest who they might be. I want you to concentrate on exercising and eating in moderation.

The National Task Force on the Prevention and Treatment of Obesity (NTFPTO) published a report reviewing the safety and efficacy of weight loss medications. They researched all of the relating studies that were published from 1966 through 1996. The three classes of drugs studied were 1) appetite suppressants/satiety increasers, such as amphetamines, fenfluramine and dexfenfluramine (Redux), 2) drugs that reduce the absorption of nutrients, such as Orlistat (experimental only), and 3) metabolism increasers, such as ephedrine and caffeine.

"*Only one* long-term, controlled study documenting the safety and efficacy of the fenfluramine-phentermine combination has been published" (NTFPTO 1996). This study was consistent with the current thought that obesity does not respond well to short-term intervention.

Although patients usually lose weight at first, the loss tends to plateau in six months and in some cases reverse despite continued drug therapy. Additionally, side effects have been reported.

"Until more data are available, pharmacotherapy *cannot* be recommended for routine use in obese individuals . . ." (NTFPTO 1996). Many people, including those with cardiovascular disease, liver problems, and children should not use weight loss drugs anyway. For them and others, the drugs are contraindicated (known to be risky).

I just (July 1997) started hearing about another study that showed Phen-Fen (see below) caused heart valves to deteriorate, which led to congestive heart failure. The test subjects, whose valves went bad, required surgery to fix the valves.

Phen-Fen (Fastin and Pondimin)

Phentermine and fenfluramine were the hottest combination in 1996, in terms of weight loss medications. As stated above, their purpose is to decrease the appetite and provide a feeling of fullness. Their potential side effects include nervousness, irritability, insomnia, constipation, dizziness, decreased sense of fatigue, dry mouth, diarrhea, abdominal pain, short-term memory loss, and pulmonary hypertension—a fatal disease (Wein 1997).

As with diets, although the drugs may cause weight loss, weight gain usually occurs after one stops taking the medication.

One weight loss program claims, "Fastin is an appetite suppressant and may act as a stimulant. Pondimin effects [sic] certain chemicals in the brain, which control eating behavior. Both medications taken together are much more effective than either alone. Side effects usually are minimal—the most common being dry mouth. Our experience is that most patients can take these medications without significant side effects." Significant to whom? They recommend the medications be used in conjunction with light exercise and a low-carbohydrate diet, specifically the soup diet. See chapter 2 for soup diet analysis. Also, people should be exercising as much as they are able and consuming about 58% of their total daily Calories in carbohydrates.

Another doctor advertises "permanent and rapid results." Permanent results have not been proven and rapid is not safe.

As of the 2005 update of this book, Phen-Fen is no longer available because of the many cases of pulmonary hypertension. Those of you who were skeptical of Phen-Fen's claims and waited until further studies were published, before trying this product, deserve a pat on the back.

When Phen-Fen was growing in popularity, one of my clients asked me if I thought that it would be alright if she took it. I said, "I've never heard of it before" and "NO! Wait about five years until after you hear about a drug before you try it, which will give researchers more time to discover side effects."

Another client, an endocrinologist, asked me if I thought that it would be alright if she prescribed Phen-Fen to her patient who was morbidly obese and diabetic, and advised (by another doctor) not to exercise due to a severe back injury. I said, "I don't know anything about that medicine" and "NO! I recommend intense nutritional intervention. A lot can be accomplished by just changing his diet."

Fortunately, both clients took my suggestions.

Redux

Similar to Fen-Phen, Redux (dexfenfluramine) decreases appetite and provides a feeling of fullness. It, too, carries side effects of dry mouth, fatigue, diarrhea, abdominal pain, short-term memory loss and pulmonary hypertension.

There are always weight loss drugs either on the market or waiting to be approved. No matter what they claim, let researchers study any given drug for many years, after FDA approval, and before you try it. Impatient people can die, including those who died from pulmonary hypertension after taking either Fen-Phen or Redux.

Always implement lifestyle changes, first.

I hope that I have discouraged you from taking weight loss medicine.

Plastic Surgery

Suction-assisted lipectomy, a form of plastic surgery, is a procedure that takes anywhere from thirty minutes to several hours in an outpatient setting. A cannula, or small pointed instrument, is placed in the problem area(s) where the surrounding fat and some fluids are vacuumed.

"Liposuction can enhance your appearance and your self-confidence, but it won't necessarily change your looks to match your ideal, or cause other people to treat you differently. Before you decide to have surgery, think carefully about your expectations and discuss them with your surgeon" (ASPRS 1994). In other words, the surgery will not help you to look like a model or a movie star whom you have been admiring.

"The best candidates are those who are of relatively normal weight but have pockets of excess fat in particular areas. You should be physically healthy, psychologically stable, and realistic in your expectations. Most important, having firm, elastic skin will result in a better final contour. (Hanging skin won't reshape to your body's new contours, and may require an additional procedure to surgically remove the excess skin. This procedure will leave visible scars.)" (ASPRS 1994). Most people probably do not realize this. When you have taken the fat away, the skin does not magically shrink to the new size of your body. Since your skin has been stretched out for so many years by excess fat, it has lost its elasticity. Doctors can easily get you back into their office for yet another surgery, because who wants hanging skin? Also, I doubt that the "best candidates" are the most common candidates. I am sure that there are plenty of obese people who are being accepted as patients, before being told to exercise and eat well. And if someone has a healthy percentage of body fat, but does not like his or her pockets of excess fat, should they take the risk that every surgery holds?

". . . In rare instances, the procedure may cause severe trauma, particularly when multiple or very extensive areas are suctioned at one time. Other infrequent, but possible, complications include fluid accumulation (which must be drained) and injury to the skin. Although serious complications are infrequent, infection or excessive fluid loss can lead to severe illness" (NTFPTO 1996) or death.

Prozac

Prozac is an anti-depressant, which has been wrongly prescribed to overweight people. I have a client whose doctor put her on the drug, because she had high blood pressure. The doctor said that Prozac would help curb her appetite, since the drug has had that side effect. If my client's appetite is curbed, her weight will drop and along with it her blood pressure, the doctor concluded.

Well, the doctor knew that my client was about to start a very regimented exercise program and healthier eating habits with a personal trainer—me—but did not give the program much of a chance. After a month-and-a-half of working with me, her blood pressure started decreasing, but the doctor started the Prozac prescription anyway. The drug did not have any positive effects and was replaced by phentermine.

Prozac, according to a well-known research psychiatrist I trained, should only be used for what it is indicated—improving the mental wellness of clinically depressed people.

Steroids

Steroids, or hormones, already occur naturally in the body. Two types—anabolic and catabolic—build up and breakdown, respectively. Anabolic is the type that is referenced most often when steroids are mentioned in a fitness context.

Ordinarily, bodybuilders—those who try to increase their muscular size for competitions—are the ones who take steroids. If you ask any given competitor if he is taking steroids, he will probably say no, whether or not he is in fact using them. They want to give the impression that their size was attained only through hard work—without a drug. Steroids can only be administered and prescribed by a physician, but are often sold illegally.

Testosterone, a male hormone, is the type of steroid that has been proven and used to increase muscle weight and strength. It is not absent of serious side effects, though, such as liver failure and hepatitis. In men, the production of sperm cells may be reduced, resulting in sterility. In women, masculine traits result (androgenic—including voice changes) along with acne and enlargement of the clitoris.

The following is the *American College of Sports Medicine Position Stand on the Use of Anabolic-Androgenic Steroids in Sports* (deVries 1994):

1. Anabolic-androgenic steroids in the presence of an adequate diet can contribute to increases in body weight, often in the lean mass compartment.
2. The gains in muscular strength achieved through high-intensity exercise and proper diet can occur by the increased use of anabolic-androgenic steroids in some individuals.
3. Anabolic-androgenic steroids do not increase aerobic power or capacity for muscular exercise.
4. Anabolic-androgenic steroids have been associated with adverse effect on the liver, cardiovascular system, reproductive system, and

psychological status in therapeutic trials and in limited research on athletes. Until further research is completed, the potential hazards of the use of the anabolic-androgenic steroids in athletes must include those found in therapeutic trials.

5. The use of anabolic-androgenic steroids by athletes is contrary to the rules and ethical principles of athletic competition as set forth by many of the sports governing bodies. The American College of Sports Medicine supports the ethical principles and deplores the use of anabolic-androgenic steroids by athletes.

In 1995 I watched a bodybuilding competition for my first time. My friend came with me and gave me information about the event specifics. This one was called a "natural" competition. I knew that it meant that the competitors would be tested for steroids, which were not allowed. My friend helped me realize that natural events are not the norm, which means normally bodybuilders are not tested for steroids. I concluded that steroid use is acceptable in the bodybuilding world. Yet like I said before, no one admits to using them.

Gastrectomy

Gastrectomy is a form of bariatric (weight loss) surgery that encompasses several means of reducing the size of the stomach. A lap-band may also be used to reduce the size of the stomach, without actually removing any of the stomach. The effectiveness stems primarily from the idea that the smaller your stomach is the less you can eat, and therefore the more likely you'll lose weight.

As you can imagine, when these surgeries were growing in popularity in the 1990s, I was very against the procedures. Then, I was fooled for a couple of years watching people I knew drop 100+ pounds in a few months. Maybe I should support the surgeries, I thought.

Then I witnessed something interesting because, of course, the people who opted for surgery didn't receive behavioral therapy. What happened? They learned how to work around their smaller stomachs. They continued to eat unhealthy while manipulating their stomachs, over time, to accept a lot of Calories. Consequently, *everyone* I observed gained back all of the lost fat weight.

In 2015 I stumbled across a letter that a medical center sent to homeowners, promoting bariatric surgery. For two reasons I almost cried when I saw it: 1) I felt like my entire career was erased, and 2) How can I get people to exercise and eat healthy when doctors are telling people to have surgery? I'm not powerful enough to go up against a medical center, though this book exists as a means for me to continue throwing punches as I exit the health and fitness industry. (I don't provide health and fitness services anymore.)

Others

"Weight Loss. New information on how to melt away fat! Lose 10, 20, 30 pounds in one month!"

"Wake up Thinner! Inches melt away while you sleep. Increases energy—tones."

Is the fat melted like butter in an air-pop popcorn machine? Just stick a slab in the metal container. When the container heats up, the fat will melt. Well, the fat does melt, but it does not disappear. Where does it go? It stays right there, waiting for you to pour it over the popcorn. Not only does it taste great but also salt sticks to it!

Is that how it works in the body? A high-tech treatment melts your fat, but then where does it go? It stays right there, waiting for you to pour it . . . Then, does salt stick to it? That would not be good. Isn't salt bad? If we have more fat melted, and therefore more salt sticking to it, would we have high blood pressure, too? Wait a minute. I thought having our fat melted was beneficial. How do we get high blood pressure out of it?

I am trying to teach you to have a light-hearted look at all of these ridiculous fitness claims. Light-hearted. Not serious. Take these claims seriously and you are bound to lose a lot of money, a lot of time when you could have been doing something truly healthy, and possibly your health in and of itself. Take these claims . . . with a grain of salt?

Do not take the easy road to wellness by having surgery or taking drugs. Exercise and eat well to achieve true health and wellbeing.

References

American Society of Plastic and Reconstructive Surgeons. 1994. Liposuction Brochure.

deVries HA, and TJ Housh. 1994. *Physiology of Exercise*. Madison: Brown & Benchmark.

National Task Force on the Prevention and Treatment of Obesity. 1996. "Long-Term Pharmacotherapy in the Management of Obesity." *JAMA* 276; 1907-15.

Wein D. 1997. "The Diet Drug Fallout." *IDEA Today* February; 50-57.

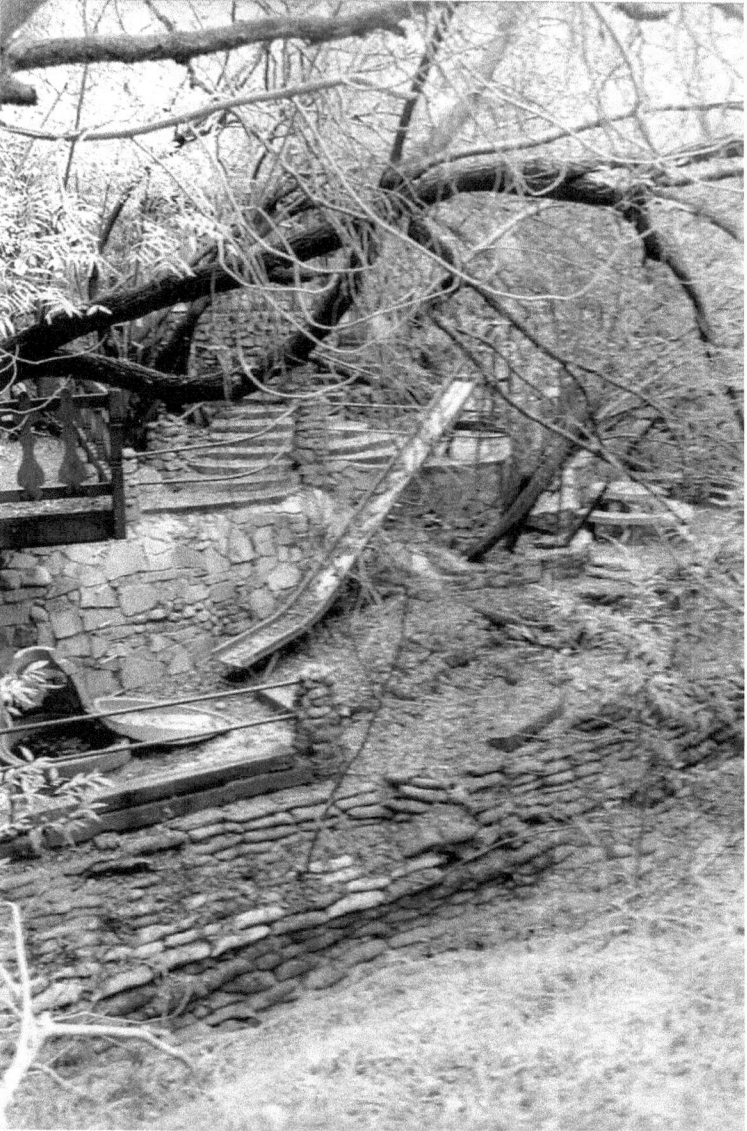

Who needs a gym when you have the ultimate playground?

Cupertino, California

CHAPTER 6

MISCELLANEOUS

The following is a list of miscellaneous products and services you might come across.

I put an asterisk after a brand name I changed for my protection. The fictitious name doesn't necessarily have anything to do with the product; it's just designed to make you laugh.

Hypnotherapy

Some hypnotherapists claim that their services can help people to lose weight. "So go ahead with hypnotherapy and achieve your goals by learning to: motivate yourself to eat what you need, understand foods, increase energy, eliminate food addictions, and get rid of negative triggers that cause emotional eating," one professional advertises.

He also states, "There will be approximately one hour a week that you have to devote to participate in a hypnotherapy session until the desired weight is achieved. Depending on your current state and where you want to aim to the average time frame necessary is between 4-10 weeks of involvement." Those statements suggest that someone could reach his weight goal within 10 weeks. Ha! Try up to two years, for some people, to achieve their weight goal.

So, does hypnotherapy work? Hypnotherapy, first of all, is not what you probably think and is not what I thought it would be. Yes, I have had it done. I thought that I would be out cold and made to do anything that the therapist wanted. No. She simply relaxed my mind and helped me to focus on what I needed to, which was retrieving a repressed memory. It worked for me, but it does not work for everyone. Does it work for weight loss? I do not know. If you are desperate for help in making permanent lifestyle changes, try it, but remember that it will act as a supplement to an exercise and healthful eating program.

Also, strive for independence. Break free from the therapy when you feel comfortable with being able to see food in a healthy perspective. Look out for the therapists who want you to stay with them for the rest of your life.

Bookracks

You may have seen people at the gym reading while on a stationary bike, stair climber, or treadmill. Do not be fooled. Although reading while exercising aerobically has no ill effects, not everyone (including me) can do it. I cannot concentrate or focus on the words. Try someone else's set-up before you invest in your own bookrack. You may find that watching television, while exercising, works better for you.

For those of you, who can read while exercising, make sure that you check your posture regularly and your perceived exertion.

Heart Rate Monitors

The best heart rate monitor that I have seen is made by Polar. A narrow strap goes around the chest and a watch-like band on the wrist. At any given moment, you can look at the "watch" to see what your pulse rate is.

It is a good idea for cardiac patients and some competitive athletes to use, but it is not a necessity for the general public. Certainly you can take your own pulse by palpating the wrist or neck, but there is usually error. Most people do not count properly.

What I am suggesting is to disregard figuring out what your pulse is at any given time and what it should be. Like I said before, there are exceptions. Instead, try using Borg's RPE (below), or rating of perceived exertion, to put a number on how intensely you are working. According to how you feel, choose the number that would best describe the intensity of your exercise:

0   Nothing at all
0.5 Very, very weak
1   Very weak
2   Weak
3   Moderate
4   Somewhat strong
5   Strong
6
7   Very strong
8
9
10 Very, very strong
*   Maximal

"Maximal" means that you are at your maximum heart rate and will either collapse, stop, or reduce the intensity. Next, decide in what number/range you want to exercise, for example 4-5. When you are exercising, ask yourself how the intensity of the workout feels. If you tell yourself "moderate," then you know to increase the intensity.

Pedometers

Pedometers offer feedback on how many steps and miles you have traveled during a walk or run, according to the stride length that you enter.

Competitive runners could benefit from one of these, during training, to ensure that they are covering the proper distance in a workout. But for the general public, it seems like just another gadget. When I design cardiovascular workouts for my clients, I focus more on time. Sure, I like to emphasize that when they become fitter they will be able to cover the same distance in a shorter period of time than at the start of their program. I just say that however much time I ask them to walk, I want them to move as fast as they can and still be able to finish. That means, if some days they need to do two hours and other days 30 minutes, the former will be a slower walk than the latter, which is fine.

As a matter of fact, it is good to alternate between low intensity long duration workouts (one hour or more) and high intensity short duration (15-59 minutes) sessions. The former can control glucose (blood sugar) levels and tolerance, decrease blood lipids (fats), and blood pressure, among other things. The latter can increase stroke volume (how much blood your heart pumps out with each beat), decrease resting heart rate, and increase $VO_{2\,max}$.

WalkinTheDog Leash

This leash can be wrapped around your waist like a belt, so that you do not have to use your hands at all.

Judging from my experiences of taking my two dogs for walks, I could not use it. If I were wearing it, I would have to become a runner. Once the dogs take off running I would have to run with them, because I would be attached to the leash at my waist. What if I took one dog at a time? Same rule applies. If you have a dog that wants to walk and does not get distracted by other animals and you want to walk, this leash might work for you. If both you and your dog want to run, then this leash could be for you, too. Just remember that you will have less control over your dog if you are not using your hands to grip a leash. Also, when my dogs get up to speeds in which I cannot keep up, I just let go of the leashes. (Do not tell the California authorities.) I am trying to warn you that there is no way that you can quickly and easily separate yourself from your dog, if you were wearing one of these leash belts.

What if another dog came up to attack you or your dog? You would not be able to get out of the way.

Skinfold Calipers

Skinfold calipers measure a fold of skin and the fat underneath it in millimeters. These are widely sold, now, as a means for people to track their percentage of body fat, which is a better number to know than weight. It signifies what percentage of your body weight is fat as opposed to lean body mass.

Taking another person's skinfold measurements is a skill that I learned in college. It takes a lot of practice to perform it correctly and knowledge of the body, specifically the muscles.

I foresee many people buying skinfold calipers and getting inaccurate results, due to inexperience. If you want to know your percentage of body fat, go to an experienced fitness evaluator. You should be able to find one in a local gym; every gym should have skinfold calipers. It only takes a few minutes to be tested and should cost relatively little, especially if you are already a gym member.

Fat-Tex Fat Analyzer*

This analyzer uses infrared technology and is placed on the biceps to measure percentage of body fat. One's gender, body weight, height, and physical activity level are entered into the machine before a percentage is given to the user.

More research is needed to perfect the equations used in this method, because large errors have been reported when compared to other, more accurate methods.

Do not get too excited or anxious about this or any similar monitor. Let the scientists research the validity of it for a few more years.

European Body Wrap

"It is a European Style shaping process that REDUCES TOXINS, FIRMS, TONES AND REDUCES INCHES. A trained technician comfortably wraps you with elastic bandages. A sea clay-like solution is used. This moderate pressure also brings the skin closer together resulting in bringing it back closer in size to its natural form."

"Lose 6 inches" in 2 hours. You may reduce cellulite and stretch marks." You will lose six inches total, as in a one-inch circumference in each of six different areas, or your whole body will be six inches less in circumference? Misleading, eh?

"No exercising or dieting." That right there should tell you that it is no good. Remember that any person or company that claims you do not need to exercise and suggests that you do not need to eat well is misleading you.

"We offer no magical claims for melting fat or redistributing tissue, we simply give your body the ability to hold a better shape by cleansing, toning and tightening your soft tissue and skin." The body can *hold* a better shape, via exercise and healthy foods, if it does not have so much fat to *hold*.

Thigh Cream

"Improve the appearance of cellulite." Why just improve the appearance of fat? Why not get rid of it? We cannot get rid of all of our fat, but by exercising and eating well, we can eliminate enough to make us healthy.

Actually, with one of my clients, I performed a little study to see if the thigh cream worked (her idea). I took a skinfold measurement on each thigh before she started using the cream and again a few weeks after she used the cream daily on just one thigh. There was no change at all on either thigh.

This same lady had had breast implant and liposuction (and probably face lift) surgeries before I met her. She was the type of person to try the easy way out toward a healthier, more youthful-looking body. Yet, those surgeries (and thigh creams) are not only very expensive but also an ineffective means toward a healthier body. And, she was still miserable. Exercise, proper nutrition, and low stress levels help the body to be and look youthful.

After training her for a year, her body fat percentage decreased only one point. Her strength training routine was pretty consistent at two times per week, but the cardiovascular exercise and nutritional habits were not good enough. These three items need to be followed at your ideal level, together, consistently. Otherwise, you may find it difficult to attain your goal.

There is soap on the market with similar claims to the thigh cream. If you see positive test results described in the New England Journal of Medicine (NEJM), then you can think that this soap is for real. If you see positive test results described in the NEJM, I will eat the soap.

Plyometrics

To enhance explosive muscular power, athletes use plyometrics. It usually involves jumping from a squat, leaping over things, and hopping. The sports for which it is useful are volleyball, basketball, and track and field, for example. Since it is such a high-intensity level of training, it should be combined with regular strength training and performed no more than two times per week.

Mel Siff concluded the following, after reviewing several studies:

"Plyometrics should be used for specialized athletic preparations, not for general fitness classes. Plyometrics should be applied with meticulous care and progression. It requires a high level of eccentric strength, explosive isometric strength and reactive skill. The so-called plyometric movements offered in commercial aerobics classes are not classical plyometric moves and should not be called plyometrics by instructors" (Monroe 1994).

An isometric contraction involves a muscle exerting force, but the muscles are not shortening and the adjacent joint is not moving. For example, if you were to try and push a wall, neither the wall would move nor your arms, but your muscles would still be exerting force.

An eccentric contraction requires a muscle to lengthen or relax slowly. For example, if you performed a push-up and then lowered yourself back to the floor slowly, your chest muscles would have to relax slowly. That is really difficult work. Doing the "easier" part of a movement extra slowly can make you a lot stronger, but usually at the price of sore muscles.

Weightlifting Belts

There has been debate as to whether or not special belts worn around the waist during lifting can prevent hernias. It is possible that studies have not shown belts to prevent hernias, because people end up lifting more weight with belts than they would without. A belt does not give you the opportunity to lift more; it enables you to lift heavy weight while supporting and stabilizing the spine.

A weightlifting belt keeps the vertebrae aligned, so that you can generate force safely. When the back is aligned, and the two sides of your back are synchronized, the risk of back injury decreases.

Wear a belt during exercises where you push weight above your head while seated or standing, and for squatting and leg pressing movements. Keep the belt fitted snugly during the set.

In between sets, the belt should be loosened to enhance blood flow and encourage the back muscles to do some work. If you have the belt tight always, the back muscles may become weak from always having help.

Make sure to have lower back and abdominal exercises in your routine to strengthen your trunk supporters (core). This will help to prevent injuries while doing everyday activities without a belt.

Pound-A-Patch*

Stick Pound-A-Patch over your mouth and replace every 24 hours. Weight loss is guaranteed, because you won't be able to eat—ever!

A client and I made that up.

Yoga

Yoga involves stretches for the joints and musculature of the trunk, while meditating and concentrating on mental wellness. Yoga offers mind relaxation, which everyone needs, but includes some movements that are unsafe to a traditionalist's mind.

For example, lunge stretches are done with the front knee over the front toes. Remember that that position can overstretch the knee ligaments. Also, the head is tilted back past the neutral position in some poses.

If you do yoga, be careful. Stretch without pain, keep your head in its neutral position, and keep your front knee over your ankle during a lunge. GO SLOWLY—AT YOUR LEVEL.

Choose yoga because you want to be in a meditative-type class, not solely for flexibility. A stretching class or personal trainer can provide safe stretches that offer benefits without the risk of injury.

How to Critique Research Studies

1. Make sure there was a large sample size (many people tested).
2. What was the media source? Did you read a report in a fashion magazine or the Journal of the American Medical Association (JAMA)?
3. Who sponsored the study? For example, did the makers of Medicine X sponsor the study on Medicine X? (The manufacturer would want favorable results.)
4. Have the study results been replicated by another researcher?
5. Was there a control group?
6. Did the investigation actually test what it intended to?
7. Were the test subjects chosen randomly or were they hand-picked?

As with exercise equipment, make sure that you investigate a product or service before investing in it. You might find that it is not right for *you*.

References

Monroe M. 1994. "The Year in Research." *IDEA Today* October; 41.

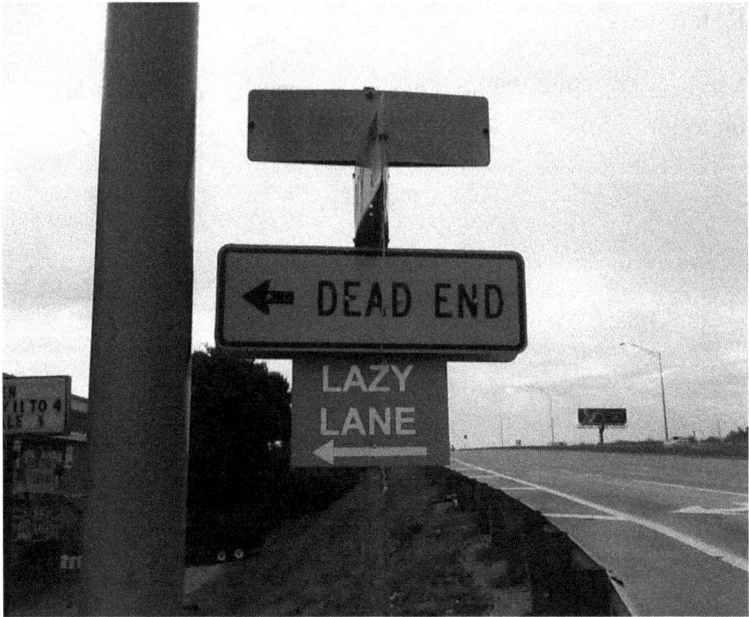

Even city and regional planners in St. Louis, Missouri, know where a sedentary lifestyle leads.

CHAPTER 7

EXERCISE AND NUTRITION MYTHS

MYTH #1:	Walking up and down hills does just as much good as walking on flat ground.
FACT #1:	Walking up and down hills, or variable terrain training, provides a means for walkers to elevate their heart rates and reap the benefits of high-intensity exercising without running. Walking down hill, slowly, eliminates the "uselessness" of declines, increases muscle strength, and reduces skeletal impact.
MYTH #2:	Running is better than walking.
FACT #2:	Anything is better than sitting. Running and walking offer excellent cardiovascular workouts. If a walker, who does not like any other type of cardiovascular exercise, is told that she will not attain any results unless she runs, she probably will stop exercising altogether. Do which exercise you like best, because anything—as long as it's safe—is better than being sedentary.

MYTH #3:   Do lots of sit-ups to make your tummy
            smaller.

FACT #3:   The sit-ups myth, a type of spot reducing,
            suggests that exercising certain muscles will
            help to reduce fat in that area. False. First of
            all, sit-ups hurt your lower back by
            imparting excessive compression force on
            the spine. Crunches (half sit-ups/roll-ups)
            are a safe alternative. Crunches, a strength-
            training exercise, increase abdominal muscle
            strength and endurance—not reduce fat.
            Strength training and cardiovascular exercise
            can help you to lose fat all over *indirectly*
            and *directly*, respectively. By
            exercising/toning the abdominal muscles,
            the waist circumference may decrease
            without decreasing abdominal fat.

MYTH #4:   The best type of equipment to use is a cross-
            country skier.

FACT #4:   The best type is that which is well-made and
            will be used by *you*.

MYTH #5:   Morning is the best time to exercise.

FACT #5:   The best time to exercise is when you will
            do it.

MYTH #6:   When doing bench press (chest exercise),
            bounce the barbell off of your chest.

FACT #6:   Bouncing the barbell off of your chest can
            break a rib and shows lack of control. When
            you lack control, you do not allow your
            muscles to work hard and you increase the
            chance of injury.

MYTH #7:   During strength training, hold your breath on
            exertion to help with the effort.

FACT #7:   Holding your breath on exertion, called the
            Valsalva Maneuver (VM), is the same as
            what we do when trying to have a bowel
            movement. Get the picture? You didn't want
            the picture? Anyway, it is very important to
            exhale on exertion, especially during
            weightlifting. Otherwise, your blood
            pressure will elevate more than it normally
            would during exercise, possibly resulting in
            an aneurysm (ballooning or bursting of an
            artery). Also, the VM may cause a hernia, a
            protrusion of a structure through the tissue
            that normally contains it.

MYTH #8:   Move in the whole range of motion when strength training.

FACT #8:   That practice is the general rule, but there are two cases when you would not. First, do not move a joint to an extent where muscle tension is lost, i.e., when the muscle can relax completely. For example, bringing dumbbells to the level of your chest, then down to your thighs (arm curls), can lose muscle tension if your elbows get a chance to straighten completely. Second, do not move a joint to an extent that you might injure it. For example, doing full squats (going from a standing position to bringing your rear near your heels) puts a tremendous amount of stress on the knees. It is safer and much more effective to go from standing to where your thighs are parallel to the floor, like sitting in a chair.

MYTH #9:   Use fast movements when weightlifting.

FACT #9:   Weight training movements need to be slow and controlled to ensure that the muscles are working hard and to prevent injury. If you want to achieve muscle endurance, just do more repetitions.

MYTH #10:   Arch your back during weightlifting, if necessary, to help move the weight.

FACT #10:   Arching your back puts a tremendous amount of stress on it. Do not ever do it. It means that the weight you are using is too heavy.

MYTH #11: Wear ankle/wrist weights or carry dumbbells during cardiovascular exercise to get your heart rate up.

FACT #11: Doing so changes your gait and puts too much stress on your joints.

MYTH #12: While doing squats, put a block of wood under your heels to make it easier.

FACT #12: People who practice this habit have tight Achilles tendons (lowest part of calf, above heel) and put a lot of stress on their knees. When the heels are elevated, the knees are forced to move forward over the ankles, causing knee damage. I am not sure why people don't just stretch their calves, rather than avoiding the limitation.

MYTH #13: You shouldn't eat right before exercising.

FACT #13: You should not exercise on a full or empty stomach. When the stomach is full during exercise, the digestive system and the exercising muscles compete for blood supply (and therefore oxygen). Usually the exercising muscles win, but do not attain as much blood as if the stomach were only partly full; this makes for a difficult exercise session. Also, the muscles winning means that digestion will be much less effective than normal. There is no harm in eating right before exercising if your stomach was empty and a small portion was consumed. The food can provide energy for the workout.

MYTH #14:   If you don't sweat, you're not working hard enough.

FACT #14:   Everyone sweats when they exercise and even at rest; you just do not always see it, because the air (if dry enough) picks up the moisture. Also, a woman's body core temperature has to elevate a degree higher than a man's does, before she will start to sweat. Men usually sweat more than women do anyway, because they have a higher metabolism. You do not have to break a sweat to reap the benefits of exercise.

MYTH #15:   Take a stretch as far as you can.

FACT #15:   When you stretch, do not hold a position that hurts. Stretch to a point that feels comfortable, or else you may create tiny tears in the muscle.

MYTH #16:   It does not matter if you keep gaining and losing weight.

FACT #16:   Constant weight gain/loss, or weight cycling, usually occurs from dieting. Some research suggests that weight cycling does not create a permanent disadvantage to losing weight the next time one tries. Every client I trained who had a history of dieting required a large time commitment to exercise. Although I have not run clinical trials, I believe that the more one diets on and off, the more difficult it will be to lose the weight correctly. Anyway, what weight cycling definitely can cause includes cardiovascular morbidity and mortality, depression, cancer, and stress.

MYTH #17:   A high-carbohydrate diet should be eaten the night before a long exercise session (lasting more than two hours).

FACT #17:   Have you heard of "hitting the wall?" It occurs when a person's body, during exercise, makes a major switch from burning mostly carbohydrates to mostly fat. Since fat requires more oxygen to burn than carbohydrates, one feels extremely sluggish when the switch occurs. If you have some fat in your diet prior to a long exercise session, the body will choose a relatively high percentage of fat as a fuel from the start, sparing high-carbohydrate use. You should want fat chosen as a fuel, because there is so much available, and the body does not try to limit its use like it does carbohydrates.

MYTH #18:   Weight-bearing exercises must be done to increase bone density.

FACT #18:   You need to ensure dense bones to prevent osteoporosis, a disease of porous bones that leads to fractures. Exercise is recommended to increase bone density, but it does not have to be weight bearing, like walking, skating, skiing, running. Non-weight-bearing exercises, such as swimming, biking, and stairclimbing are beneficial, too. Weight bearing means that you are supporting your body during aerobic exercise, rather than having a machine or water support you. Weight bearing exercise does not refer to weight lifting (strength training). Although all forms of exercise can increase bone density, the most beneficial is strength training, because it puts the most amount of stress (positive) on the muscles and therefore bones. The second most effective is weight-bearing exercise, and third is non-weight-bearing exercise. Remember one last point: if you *only* walk, you will increase bone density in the legs and back *only*. The arms will not benefit unless they are exercised, too, as with swimming and strength training.

MYTH #19:   Some thin people have 0% body fat.

FACT #19:   Everyone has some body fat, or else they would be dead, because the brain is all fat (and water). Essential body fat for men is 3% and for women 10%. Healthy is 10-15% and 15-20%, respectively, and obese is 25% or higher and 30% or higher, respectively.

MYTH #20:   Exercise machines can give you an accurate display of how many Calories you are burning.

FACT #20:   Step onto a treadmill, and the first thing it will ask you is how much you weigh. It wants to give you a reading, during exercise, of how many Calories you are burning. The amount will not be accurate, because it does not know your percentage of body fat or how trained you are—two key factors in determining metabolism. If you do decide to enter your weight, consider the reading an approximation.

MYTH #21:   Exercise can enhance your sex life.

FACT #21:   I will not argue with that one.

MYTH #22:   Everyone gains at least a few pounds over the holidays.

FACT #22:   Some people make exercise a priority during the holidays and eat in moderation and, therefore, do not gain weight.

MYTH #23:   It's impossible to eat healthy at restaurants.

FACT #23:   Restaurants want your business. They know
             that if you do not like or get what you
             ordered, you may not return. Also, more and
             more establishments are making an effort to
             have some, if not all, healthy choices. You
             are the patron who is paying and you are the
             one who needs to be healthy, so special
             order if necessary and ask lots of questions.
             You should know exactly how your food is
             prepared and what the ingredients are—a
             person with allergies would. You can, too!
             In some places, the chef will even come out
             to your table to consult you.

MYTH #24:   Stretches must be done before exercising.

FACT #24:   Stretches do not have to be done before
            every type of exercising, especially if the
            muscles are cold. Since stretching cold
            muscles can create microscopic tears in the
            tissue, at least five minutes of warming the
            muscles must be done first. You could walk,
            jog, or do a low intensity of the activity you
            are about to perform. Stretching does not
            have to be done before weight lifting and
            most cardiovascular exercises as long as you
            start slowly. If the cardiovascular exercise
            were long in duration and/or a competition, I
            would recommend stretching first. Sports
            such as golf, tennis, soccer, baseball, and
            others with ballistic (quick, reflexive,
            jarring, bouncing) movements also require
            stretching first (after a warm-up). The most
            important time to stretch is after exercising,
            when the muscles are very warm.

MYTH #25:   It's good to mix up your strength training routine by doing different exercises each session.

FACT #25:   The strength training routine should have variety to keep the muscles and the mind stimulated. Changing it about every three months meets that need. Changing the exercises frequently does not allow the muscles enough time to learn. Providing a muscle with the same movement from session to session gives it a chance to learn and adapt to the stress (positive). When the muscle is consistently challenged with the same movement at higher intensities, it increases in size and strength to accomplish the task. It is the result of learning and adapting.

MYTH #26:   If you stop exercising, your muscles will turn to fat.

FACT #26:   Muscles cannot turn to fat. Fat cannot turn to muscle. These two are completely separate tissues. One cannot turn into the other. When you stop exercising, the enlarged muscles atrophy, or decrease in size, because they are no longer challenged. When muscle tissue is lost, the metabolism decreases, because there is less tissue requiring energy. If you continue to consume the same amount of Calories as before, a positive energy balance results, and therefore more fat is stored. People usually gain fat at the cessation of exercise, because of consuming unneeded Calories.

125

CONCLUSION

When driving the highway to wellness, steer clear of quackery; a lot exists. The quackery can stem from exercise products, nutrition, fitness professionals, the media, and medical treatment. If a product or service advertises fast or easy-to-obtain results, the fountain of youth, or a fixed-term program, it will not work. As for exercise, no effective weight loss program provides such choices.

As discussed earlier, many videotapes, books, and equipment manufacturers, among others, market the "perfect" workout. Even if the source is credible, it cannot possibly give you a <u>personalized</u> program without knowing <u>you</u>! Remember that these items are *mass*-produced. Do you really think that there are thousands of people with the *same* exercise goals and the *same* medical history as you? These are the facts that a personal fitness trainer needs to consider.

After obtaining physician approval to commence an exercise program, consult a personal fitness trainer in your area. He should hold at least a bachelor of science degree in an exercise-related field. *This* route should be taken to get your personalized workout.

Good luck deciphering future claims and remember to use skepticism. It could save you a lot of money and preserve your health.

ABOUT THE AUTHOR

Entrepreneur and satirist Jeanne "Bean" Murdock brings a new approach to comedy, fusing observational humor with health and fitness knowledge. Performing on roller skates where she can, her improvised physical comedy is one that has never been done before. Jeanne's sassy, naive perspective wins audiences' attention, demanding that "the show must go on."

Jeanne's on-stage alter ego is quite different from the straight-laced persona that people were used to seeing when she taught health and fitness and business. When Jeanne steps up to the microphone, her otherwise compassionate approach disappears.

Originally from Cupertino, California, Jeanne was given the nickname Bean, in third grade, by her next-door neighbor, simply because it rhymed with Jeanne. She studied physical education at California Polytechnic State University in San Luis Obispo, and then started BEANFIT HEALTH AND FITNESS SERVICES in 1992. Three years later, Jeanne was diagnosed with celiac disease, a condition that she included in her teachings. For 22 years she was a health and fitness professional who also happened to be a comedian. Now, she is a comedian who happens to be a health and fitness expert.

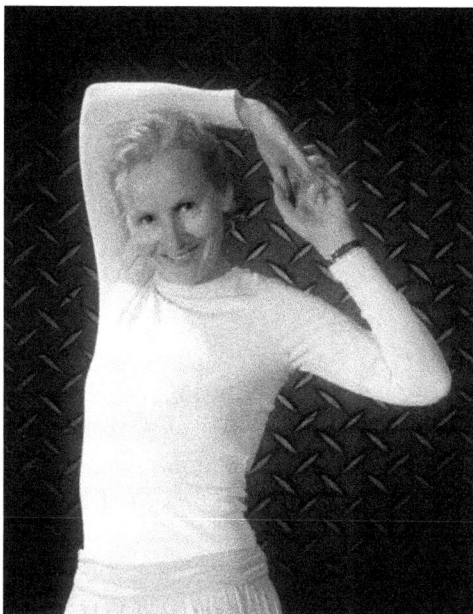

Image by Jim Tyler, edited by Greg Heller

Qualifications:

--Bachelor of Science in Physical Education
concentration: Commercial/Corporate Fitness
Cal Poly State University, San Luis Obispo.

--Undergraduate Nutrition Coursework Completed
San Diego State University.

Questions? Comments? Please feel free to write or call
Jeanne "Bean" Murdock anytime at:

PO Box 1083
Paso Robles, CA 93447
Phone: 408-203-7643
Website: www.JeanneMurdock.com
E-mail: laugh@JeanneMurdock.com

Other books by Jeanne "Bean" Murdock:
*The Every Excuse in the Book Book: How to Benefit from
Exercising, by Overcoming Your Excuses*
*Successful Dating at Last! A Workbook for Understanding
Each Other*
*It's Hard to Find Good Help These Days: A Customer
Service Manual for Businesses*

www.ingramcontent.com/pod-product-compliance
Lightning Source LLC
Chambersburg PA
CBHW070251290326
41930CB00041B/2448